Not Just Any Department
of Family Medicine

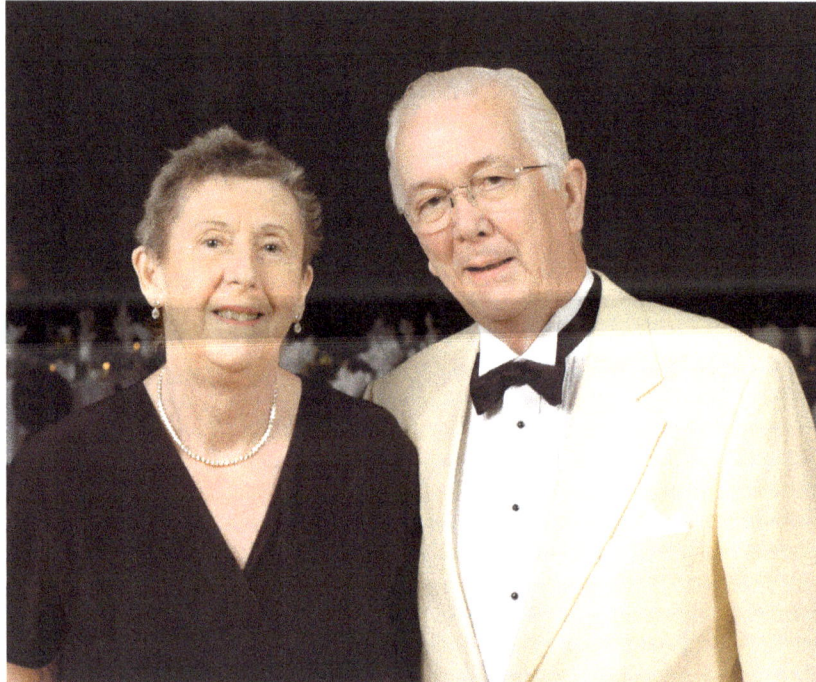

This book is dedicated to Terence C. Davies, MD, and
S. Margaret Davies, MD, who are without a doubt the
founding parents and continuing conscience of the University
of Michigan Department of Family Medicine community.

NOT JUST ANY DEPARTMENT OF FAMILY MEDICINE

Telling the Story of the First Forty Years of the
University of Michigan Department of Family Medicine

Kent J. Sheets, PhD

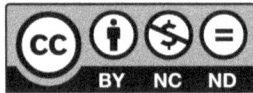

Published in the United States of America by
Michigan Publishing

DOI: 10.3998/mpub.9939973

ISBN 978-1-60785-454-8 (paper)

ISBN 978-1-60785-455-5 (e-book)

An imprint of Michigan Publishing, Maize Books serves the publishing needs of the University of Michigan community by making high-
quality scholarship widely available in print and online. It represents a
new model for authors seeking to share their work within and beyond
the academy, offering streamlined selection, production, and distri-
bution processes. Maize Books is intended as a complement to more
formal modes of publication in a wide range of disciplinary areas.

http://www.maizebooks.org

Contents

Foreword

In 1978, when the University of Michigan Department of Family Medicine was established as the Department of Family Practice (DFP), the world was very different. The first Apple computer was being tested. Cell phones had not yet been conceived, let alone apps like FaceTime. IBM was one of the biggest companies in the world, while Google, Microsoft, and Amazon were not even concepts.

In the health care arena, health maintenance organizations (HMOs) were in their infancy, diagnosis-related groups (DRGs) had not been developed, and physicians and hospitals were paid whatever they billed. The specialty of family practice was less than a decade old. And the University of Michigan Medical Center was configured quite differently from today's Michigan Medicine.

It was in that milieu that a group of visionary family physicians, led by George A. Dean, MD, worked with the state legislature until it agreed to leverage the University of Michigan to establish the DFP. Thus, five intrepid faculty pioneers, under the leadership of inaugural chair Terrence C. Davies, MD, began a department at the University of Michigan, one of the world's premier institutions. They likely had no idea they were launching what would become one of the world's top family medicine programs. The origin story of this program is detailed in this book, written by a faculty member, Kent J. Sheets, PhD, who joined the department in 1982.

The University of Michigan is special. I was told this when I came here in 1989, though I admit I was skeptical. To my delight, I've come to appreciate that "special something," to perceive it in so many ways, and I am honored to be part of the special world that is family medicine at the University of Michigan. *Not Just Any Family Medicine Department* is a tribute to all who have been a part of this program over the past forty years, as well as to those who will join it.

This is a story of the highs and lows (mostly highs!) of being a countercultural department and of the incredible people who have helped make the department so successful. When people ask me what makes Michigan so great, the answer is easy. It's the people. We have the real dream team (faculty *and* staff), and we never lose sight of why we're here—to help patients and their families be healthy, whether by direct patient care, teaching others to be the best doctors possible, or finding new ways of providing better care.

Another reason we've done so well is that we stand on the shoulders of giants. Dr. Sheets highlights many of these giants in this book—the founding fathers who refused to take "no" for an answer when pushing for this specialty to be included at the University of Michigan; the first chair, Dr. Davies, who overcame great odds to get the program started at such a highly prestigious medical school; and his successor, Thomas L. Schwenk, MD, whose vision and leadership grew the program into a top-ten department. There are other faculty and staff that Dr. Sheets highlights, as well as many who haven't been mentioned because of lack of space. The giants before us sacrificed, persevered, and made sure that this program succeeded. It's not an accident that it exemplifies the "Leaders and Best" theme in the school fight song. There are high expectations for those at Michigan. The people—who not only are brilliant but work together and pull for each other—and the guidance and commitment of the giants who have shown the way have allowed the Department of Family Medicine to succeed in meeting those expectations.

Many who know me are aware that in many ways, I'm a former jock who is still one at heart. As our faculty will confirm, I continue to believe in and emphasize "the team, the team, the team." It was the theme of my chalk talk when I was one of the final candidates for the chair position in 2012. It is why I brought Lloyd Carr, the coach of our 1997 national championship football team, to talk to the department at a State of the Department Address (SODA) event. And it is why I brought Carol Hutchins, the coach of our 2005 national championship softball team, to talk at another SODA event about the importance of teamwork. I'm proud to say that people at the University of Michigan really do embrace this concept. We work together very closely, and we all have each other's backs. When anyone needs coverage for a shift or a precepting session or when there is a family emergency, someone else always steps up. When there's a need for someone to review a manuscript, we will do it for each other. When someone is stuck with a difficult problem, there's always someone else who will help solve it. We celebrate our successes and support each other during our losses (departmentally or individually). This type of environment reflects the culture our first department chairs, Drs. Davies and Schwenk, developed, and I thank them for this environment of camaraderie, caring, and support. This is who we are and part of why we are a special place.

Thus, it's no wonder that the medical students rate us so highly year after year; that we have so many applicants for our residency spots; that we're able to continue recruiting talented new faculty members; that patient demand for our family physicians is so overwhelming; and that we are so successful in competing for grants and publishing groundbreaking improvements in care.

Since October 2016, our executive committee has put together an ambitious, strategic plan designed to ensure that the Department of Family Medicine remains a special place as well as the "Leaders and Best" in the new evolving health care paradigms. Most importantly, the plan focuses on making sure we do what we all came here to do—provide the best possible care for our patients and their families. The plan not only supports our three missions (teaching, patient care, and research), but it also aims to maximize our "joy of work," enhance our diversity, and provide for ongoing faculty development. I'm excited and optimistic to see this play out and remain very confident that we will succeed.

I hope you enjoy reading this book as much as I did.

Here's to the next forty! Go Blue!

Philip Zazove, MD

Acknowledgments

I am extremely grateful for all the assistance and wisdom I have received throughout the preparation of this book. In trying to list all the relevant people, I am bound to leave someone out, so I apologize in advance for any omissions.

Inside the department, R. Dale Lefever, PhD, and Sandra M. Genske provided close scrutiny and constructive feedback in reviewing each draft. Outside the department, my friend of over thirty years, R. Clark Malcolm, PhD, brought his expertise as an editor of nineteen books to his role of editing book number twenty. He and his wife will receive a trip to Gettysburg National Military Park in partial payment for his services.

The staff members of the Center for the History of Family Medicine in Leawood, Kansas, were instrumental in helping me locate original source materials, as were staff members of the University of Michigan Bentley Historical Library.

John J. Frey III, MD, was the person who initially encouraged me to pursue this project, and his counsel was a positive reminder of its purpose throughout the process.

Numerous people were interviewed for this book. All the interviewees and interviewers are listed among the notes and sources.

There are long lists of people, awards, and numbers included in the appendices. These lists were compiled, updated, and/or typed by Blythe A. Bieber, Andrea R. Murawa, Deborah A. Wright, Amy C. St. Amour, and Sandra Genske.

All the photographs and other images used in this book were taken or created by individuals working as employees of the University of Michigan Department of Family Practice or Department of Family Medicine (depending on the year) or by people who were contracted by the department to take photographs strictly for the use of the department.

Specific individuals whose photographs are used include James M. Cooke, MD; D. Stephanie Dascola; Damon L. Holmes; Kristen H. Ochomogo; and Kent J. Sheets, PhD. Michigan Photography and its predecessors, including the University of Michigan Information Services, were contracted to take photos (particularly the black-and-white photos from the early years) for various departmental marketing or communication efforts.

The timelines were based on several existing timelines created by group efforts of previously mentioned individuals.

Finally, I am honored to acknowledge the contributions of the three individuals who have served as my department chairs and colleagues throughout my academic career at the University of Michigan. Terence C. Davies, MD; Thomas L. Schwenk, MD; and

Philip Zazove, MD, contributed paper and electronic source materials that were critical to compiling the story of the University of Michigan Department of Family Medicine. They were also among the interviewees. I could not have conducted this project without their full cooperation and support.

I am forever indebted to all the people listed above and numerous others who have contributed to this project, especially Patrick Goussy at Michigan Publishing Services, and Elvis Ramirez, Jamie Harrison, Tim Durning, and Lauren Conkling at Scribe Inc., who made my manuscript into a well-designed and meticulously edited book. Thank you all.

Kent J. Sheets, PhD
October 19, 2017

NOT JUST ANY DEPARTMENT OF FAMILY MEDICINE

Telling the Story of the First Forty
Years of the University of Michigan
Department of Family Medicine

Kent J. Sheets, PhD

Preface

This book is being written midway through the fortieth year of the existence of the University of Michigan Department of Family Medicine in anticipation of the official celebration of its anniversary on March 1, 2018.

In an effort to make disclaimers up front, I acknowledge that some things will be given less coverage than people with an investment in a particular time frame or department mission might view as appropriate. That is the nature of trying to document such a dynamic and highly successful organization.

One thing has become clear in doing the research to prepare this historical account. There is value to having contemporaneous written materials (letters, committee reports, memos, printed email messages, etc.) to use to confirm memories. The old adage of "don't let the truth get in the way of a good story" frequently came to mind and likely will continue to come to mind as people read this history over the years.

The goal of this book is to inform the reader how the department got here in the first place, how it encountered and survived some setbacks, the highlights of what it has done in forty years, and what its members anticipate for the future.

In some ways, this is the story of a very successful small business, one that has been operating in the midst of the University of Michigan, one of the most prestigious public universities in the country—if not the world—which celebrated its own two-hundred-year anniversary in 2017.

As for the title, *Not Just Any Department of Family Medicine*, Horace W. Davenport, a distinguished professor of physiology at the University of Michigan Medical School, wrote a history that was titled *Not Just Any Medical School: The Science, Practice, and Teaching of Medicine at the University of Michigan, 1850–1941*. The title of this book pays homage to Professor Davenport and his work of a much larger scope while focusing on one specific department, which has existed since March 1, 1978.

In helping me finish this book, Dr. Zazove wrote a succinct account of why this department is not just any family medicine department and why we will carry the lessons of the previous forty years into the future.

Nearly two hundred individuals have served as faculty members in the forty years since our humble beginnings, all of whom have contributed in their diverse yet special individual ways. They have constituted, in Dr. Zazove's words, "our dream team"—a team that has excelled in the clinical arena; in the teaching of students, residents, fellows, and faculty; in cutting-edge research; and in multiple leadership roles. This team has clearly exemplified the motto of the University of Michigan: "Leaders and Best."

1

1966 to 1978
Setting the Stage

The decades of the 1960s and 1970s in the United States were periods of notable social, political, and economic change. Medicine and medical education were among the institutional areas affected by changes that pervaded those turbulent eras. Movements at the national, statewide, and local levels eventually led to the establishment of the University of Michigan Department of Family Practice (DFP), beginning on March 1, 1978. This is the story of that department.

No individual event, person, or organization led to the creation of this department; rather, a collection of events, forces, and decisions at the local, state, and national levels coalesced to bring about the decision to establish the department. Local family physicians in Washtenaw County and their colleagues in the Michigan Academy of Family Physicians (MAFP) were powerful voices, as were national commissions and reports during the evolution of the traditional general practitioner into the family physician.

At the state level, general practice was also beginning to evolve into family practice when a combination of general practitioners, family physicians, and insightful state legislators joined forces to initiate legislation and funding to support the development of academic departments of family practice at the three state allopathic medical schools: Wayne State University, Michigan State University (MSU), and the University of Michigan.

Two national reports from the American Medical Association in 1966—the Millis Commission Report[1] and the Willard Report[2]—led to further support for family practice as a specialty, including the establishment of residency training programs.

Among other activities at the national level, the Society of Teachers of Family Medicine (STFM) was established in 1967 to represent the academic interests of the growing movement. In February 1969, the American Board of Family Practice became the twentieth specialty board recognized by the American Board of Medical Specialties.

Finally, the American Academy of General Practice, originally established in 1947, changed its name to the American Academy of Family Physicians (AAFP) in October 1971 to reflect changes going on in primary care practice across the country.

In Lansing, the Michigan State Legislature passed a resolution in the spring of 1971 urging the establishment of departments of family practice at Wayne State University, MSU, and the University of Michigan.

Senate Concurrent Resolution No. 47 included the following:

> WHEREAS, It seems apparent that correction of this gross disparity must be made at its source—the schools of medicine which provide the great majority of physicians who take up practice in Michigan—and that, in order to alleviate the situation, these schools must strongly emphasize the great need for and desirability of family practice; now therefore be it
>
> RESOLVED BY THE SENATE (the House of Representatives concurring), That the three schools of medicine in Michigan, located at the University of Michigan, Michigan State University, and Wayne State University, are hereby urged to establish Departments of Family Practice, to encourage the development of family physicians; and be it further
>
> RESOLVED, That copies of this resolution be transmitted to the head of each of the above-mentioned schools of medicine.
>
> Adopted by the Senate, April 7, 1971.
>
> Adopted by the House of Representatives, May 14, 1971.[3]

In Washtenaw County, a group of family physicians met with representatives from the leadership of the University of Michigan Hospital, St. Joseph Mercy Hospital, and Chelsea Community Hospital in 1971 and 1972 to develop and submit a proposal for a Washtenaw County family practice residency program that would be shared across the three hospitals. The proposal was denied in 1973 by the accreditation review group, but the meetings between these groups helped establish initial relationships among these institutions that would pay off several years later.

A Grass Roots Description of the Experience of Students at the Three Michigan Medical Schools

Three students enrolled in medical school in the state of Michigan in the 1970s are talking about a patient with a common condition. The Wayne State trained student says, "I have seen hundreds of patients with that problem." The Michigan State trained student says, "I can really relate to that patient and the psychosocial issues associated with having that problem." The University of Michigan trained student says, "I have read everything there is to read about that problem, but I have never actually seen a patient with that problem."

Building upon successful efforts to establish departments at Michigan State and Wayne State, the MAFP and local area family physicians continued to lobby the University of Michigan to establish a department of family practice there. A key meeting was held between MAFP representatives and the Board of Regents on February 21, 1975. MAFP leadership prepared background materials for the regents and presented these materials in person. The three primary MAFP representatives were Cecelia F. Hissong, MD, MAFP president; Robert W. Oakes, MD, MAFP president-elect; and George A. Dean, MD, MAFP vice president.

The cumulative effects of these efforts eventually led to the establishment of a "Planning Committee regarding a Family Practice Residency for the University of Michigan Medical School," as outlined in a letter written by John A. Gronvall, MD, dean of the medical school, dated October 31, 1975: "My own position is that Family Practice has now achieved status as a recognized specialty, there is demonstrated public desire that the number of Family Physicians be increased, and our own students are increasingly seeking such residency training. It is further my belief that for the University of Michigan to establish a quality training program in this discipline that can be most effectively accomplished through the establishment of a Department of Family Practice, although there are other models which other institutions have used successfully."[4]

The Residency Planning Committee (RPC) was chaired by J. Robert Willson, MD, chair of the University of Michigan Department of Obstetrics and Gynecology, and co-chaired by George A. Dean, MD, as the official representative of the MAFP. Other family practice representation was provided by Dale L. Williams, MD, a community family physician from Muskegon also involved in MAFP leadership, and Gary R. Gazella, MD, a third-year family practice resident at the Oakwood Hospital Residency Program and 1973 graduate of the University of Michigan Medical School (UMMS). A fourth-year medical student who was interviewing for family practice residency programs, Judith C. Holt, also served on the committee.

Members of the Residency Planning Committee, established October 31, 1975
J. Robert Willson, MD, chair
George A. Dean, MD, co-chair
Gary R. Gazella, MD
Roland G. Hiss, MD
Judith C. Holt, medical student
Ramon R. Joseph, MD
Charles L. Votaw, MD, PhD
Dale L. Williams, MD
Thomas L. Stern, MD, consultant from the AAFP

After a series of meetings, including consultation with key department chairs and national representatives of family practice, the committee submitted its report, stating that a "key issue, upon which the committee spent a considerable amount of time, was whether a family practice program should be constituted administratively as a department in its own right or as a division within an already established department. It is the unanimous recommendation of the committee that a Department of Family Practice be established."[5]

At the time of the completion of the RPC report, the location for the clinical site had not been finalized: "Some of the committee members believe that the program would best be located in the University Hospital. This belief is based on the perception of the importance of this new specialty of the practice of medicine. However, the committee unanimously agrees that this would be difficult to accomplish and therefore believes at this time Wayne County General Hospital is the preferred site for location of the residency."[6]

Following the submission of the RPC report in the spring of 1976, the recommendation was quickly approved by the medical school executive committee and by the Board of Regents in November of that year.

One of the members of the RPC was Charles L. Votaw, MD, PhD, associate dean for curriculum. Dr. Votaw requested a consultation from the AAFP, and Daniel J. Ostergaard, MD, assistant director of the AAFP Division of Education, came to the area on January 17, 1977. Dr. Ostergaard met with key individuals and submitted a consultation report on January 21, 1977, which included a very significant recommendation: "Chelsea Medical Clinic should be pursued as the number one possibility for a superior family practice center in a combined residency between Chelsea Community Hospital and the University of Michigan Hospital."[7]

Quickly, the medical school leadership moved forward with the establishment of a search committee for the founding chair, with Drs. Willson, Dean, and Votaw serving on that committee to provide continuity with the deliberations of the RPC. Another source of continuity was provided at the staff level as Peggy L. Alford, who was Dr. Votaw's administrative assistant, provided staff support to both the RPC and the search committee.

Key Groups/Individuals in the Era between 1966 and 1978

Washtenaw County area family physicians

Michigan Academy of Family Physicians

Michigan State Legislature

Key administrators at UMMS

John A. Gronvall, MD, dean of the medical school, 1970–82

Charles L. Votaw, MD, PhD, associate dean for curriculum

J. Robert Willson, MD, chair of the Department of Obstetrics and Gynecology

Members of the Residency Planning Committee

Daniel J. Ostergaard, MD, assistant director of the AAFP Division of Education

The total number of applicants is unrecorded, but six candidates were brought to campus for interviews and four candidates were chosen for Dean Gronvall to consider. Terence C. Davies, MD, from the University of South Alabama was among those candidates, and on October 5, 1977, he was offered the position, which he accepted on October 20, 1977. The prehistory of the University of Michigan DFP ended when a start date of March 1, 1978, was established in the negotiations between Dr. Davies and Dean Gronvall.

Many things in the history of this department are easier to appreciate many years later, while others are harder to understand given lack of sufficient documentation. Several things are readily apparent in considering what led to the approval of this new department.

The time was right in the state of Michigan and at the University of Michigan for a variety of reasons. The MAFP and state legislature played big roles, as did local family physicians, previous efforts to establish a family practice residency in the Washtenaw County, and a more formal family practice presence at the University of Michigan. As a statement from the RPC report reflects, the fact that the University wanted state funding to help build a new University Hospital certainly played a role as well: "The administrator at the University of Michigan Hospital believes that there is direct poligical [sic] pressure from the state legislature and from the people of the State of Michigan to create a family practice program. He also believes that it would be politically important to institute the program at the University Hospital in view of our plan to seek public funds for a new hospital."[8]

There were also some unreasonable expectations included in the RPC report: "The target date for initiating the residency program is July 1, 1979. At that time, it is estimated there will be 7 first year and 3 second year house officers. When fully operational there will be a total of 30 residents in the 3 years of the program."[9] In reality, it was many years before the residency program totaled thirty residents.

As another example of outsized expectations, the RPC used an external report on the potential value of the Chelsea Medical Center in terms of patient revenue to be realized by the University Hospital with numbers that were highly inflated. But the stage had been set for the incorporation of the specialty of family practice into the highly subspecialized setting of the University Michigan Hospitals.

Chapter 1 Timeline: Key Events/Individuals between 1966 and 1978

1966	American Medical Association releases national reports: Millis Commission Report and Willard Report
1967	Society of Teachers of Family Medicine (STFM) is established
1969	American Board of Family Practice is established
1971	American Academy of General Practice changes to American Academy of Family Physicians (AAFP)
1971	Michigan State Legislature approves resolutions to establish departments of family practice at the three state university allopathic medical schools

1972–73	Washtenaw County family practice residency proposal is submitted and denied
February 1975	Michigan Academy of Family Physicians (MAFP) representatives meet with Board of Regents and Dean Gronvall
October 1975	Residency planning committee is established
November 1976	Board of Regents approves Department of Family Practice
January 1977	AAFP Ostergaard Consultation Report recommends Chelsea as clinical site
October 1977	Terence C. Davies, MD, accepts offer to serve as first chair

2

1978 to 1986
Growing Pains and Crisis Management

T erence C. Davies, MD, deliberately chose the start date of March 1, 1978, so his appointment as the founding chair of the Department of Family Practice (DFP) would coincide with Saint David's Day, a national festival day in his native Wales. This reflected one of many traditions he brought with him from his Welsh and British heritage as he set about to fulfill the tasks associated with establishing a department of family practice at the University of Michigan. The first office space was on the second floor of Medical Science Building I, adjacent to animal research labs, which meant that the odors and noises from dogs and monkeys were omnipresent in the hallways and elevators that led to the space.

One of the first tasks on his to-do list was the hiring of support staff. His first decision was to build on relationships established during the work of the Residency Planning Committee (RPC) and search committee process by hiring Peggy L. Alford, an

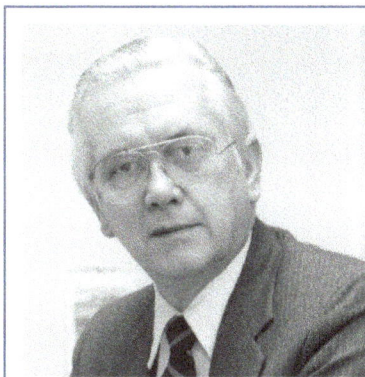

NAME: Terence C. Davies, MD
ROLE: First professor and chair of the DFP
BIO: Previously faculty at University of South Alabama and Medical University of South Carolina

Location on March 1, 1978: Ann Arbor, Michigan, starting his first day as founding chair administrative assistant to Charles L. Votaw, MD, PhD, the associate dean of curriculum in the years prior to the founding of the department. Ms. Alford was an experienced staff member of the University of Michigan Hospital and Medical School and thus brought her knowledge of the University system and others with whom Dr. Davies would be interacting as he established this new department.

Shortly thereafter, with the assistance of several key acquaintances in the medical school and the Association for American Medical Colleges (AAMC), R. Dale Lefever, PhD, was hired as the first faculty member in the position of assistant professor and director of educational development. Dr. Lefever was the associate director of the AAMC Division of Faculty Development at the time of his hiring, and prior to that, he had worked for three years in the Michigan State University (MSU) Office of Medical Education, Research, and Development. His doctoral degree was in administration and higher education. Drs. Lefever and Davies and Ms. Alford formed the core cohort of "firsts" among many firsts in this department history: first chair, first staff, and first faculty member.

One of the many fortunate developments in the history of the DFP was the selection of Chelsea as the location for the first faculty and resident outpatient clinical site, adjacent to the Chelsea Community Hospital, fifteen miles west of Ann Arbor. It is apparent from contemporaneous reports and interviewing members of the RPC that there was no interest on the part of the medical school in having the department's clinical site located in Ann Arbor, and at times, it appeared that placing it at the Wayne County General Hospital site—which was already affiliated with the medical school—was the goal. While it was not documented who made the decision to choose Chelsea as the site, the choice has worked in everyone's benefit since day one.

As administrative staff members were hired in Ann Arbor, the Chelsea site transitioned from a private practice to a University-owned practice. Many of the family physicians and other office and clinical staff remained at the site to provide continuity of care for the existing patients. The proximity to Chelsea Community Hospital also facilitated the establishment of a faculty presence in the community hospital inpatient setting during the transition from a community to academic practice model.

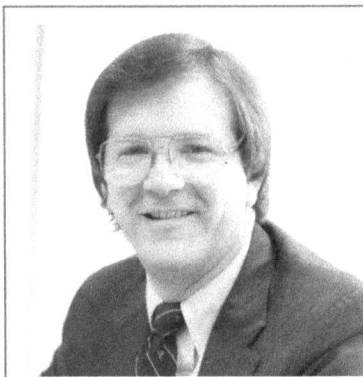

NAME: R. Dale Lefever, PhD
ROLE: First assistant professor and director of educational development
BIO: Previously at AAMC and MSU Office of Medical Education, Research, and Development

Location on March 1, 1978: Washington, DC, working for the AAMC

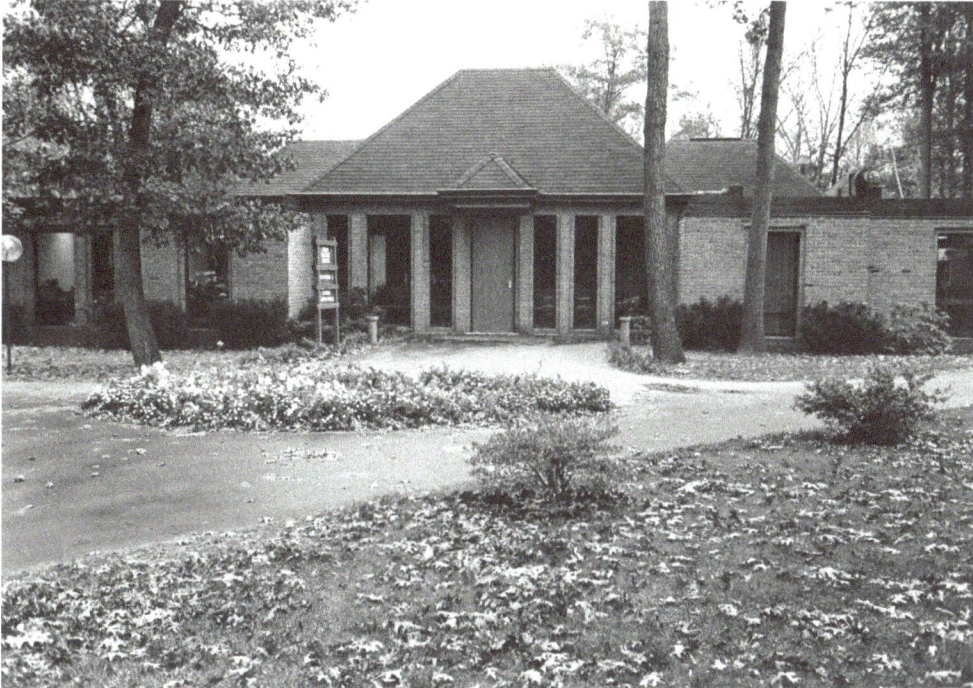

Figure 2.1. Original Chelsea Family Practice Center

Since a primary purpose for establishing the department was to add a family practice residency to the collection of residency programs in the University of Michigan system, some of Dr. Davies's first efforts were to contact people at the American Academy of Family Physicians (AAFP) and the Accreditation Council of Graduate Medical Education to determine the process and timeline for getting a new residency accredited so he could start recruiting a first group of residents. He also spoke to the chair of a department of family practice at another large midwestern public university in order to get insight from someone working in a similar environment.

One of the people that Dr. Davies spoke to at the AAFP was Daniel J. Ostergaard, MD, the assistant director of the Division of Education. In that role, Dr. Ostergaard was involved in reviewing existing family practice residency programs and consulting with hospitals and schools that were considering establishing family practice programs. Dr. Ostergaard had also conducted a consultation in January 1977, following the approval of the department by the Board of Regents in November 1976. Among his recommendations, Dr. Ostergaard highlighted the potential of Chelsea as the most appropriate site for the resident and faculty outpatient site. As another link to the AAFP, director of the AAFP Division of Education, Thomas L. Stern, MD, had served as a consultant to the RPC and made several visits to Ann Arbor during the deliberations of that committee. Dr. Davies also consulted with Dr. Stern during the early days of the department.

With this and other input, Drs. Davies and Lefever and Ms. Alford began to write the residency accreditation application document. Concurrently, they began work on a residency training grant application, which when approved and funded would provide support for faculty and staff salaries and equipment like video cameras, recorders, and one-way mirrors, which were used in training residents in the Chelsea Family Practice Center.

In July 1978, Dr. Davies submitted a progress report and planning overview to Dean Gronvall. Looking at the items identified as planning priorities for the department on July 18, 1978, it is noteworthy that few have changed since that time:

A. Stabilize and develop patient-care at the Family Practice Center for further equipping, renovating and extending of present facilities. Resolve those identified problems which are present within the Family Practice Center. Work on community relations and patient education concerning Family Practice.

B. Complete an Affiliation Agreement with the Chelsea Community Hospital.

C. Complete a curriculum proposal for the Family Practice Residency Program in collaboration with all major departments in the Medical College.

D. Seek further funding (Kellogg Foundation, HEW, etc.) for special program development.

E. Recruit needed faculty.

F. Identify and develop teaching input into the undergraduate curriculum (including individual student needs, electives and "core" curricula).

G. Further develop research goals and protocols and prioritize research ambitions.

H. Continue and develop collaborative efforts for Continuing Medical Education for Family Physicians.

I. Plan a sequence of faculty development exercises.[1]

As work proceeded on the accreditation and training grant applications, the decision was made to recruit potential members of the first class of family practice residents, who would start as interns in July 1979. A complicating factor was that it would not be known at the time that resident applicants submitted their materials to the National Residency Match Program if the new residency program had been approved by the accrediting body. In the event that the program was not accredited in time to start training residents in July 1979, Dean Gronvall agreed to help find rotating internships for the four University of Michigan Medical School (UMMS) students in the class of 1979 who chose to gamble on being the first residents in this new program.

Key Groups/Individuals between 1978 and 1986

Terence C. Davies, MD

Peggy L. Alford

R. Dale Lefever, PhD

First four residents

John A. Gronvall, MD, dean of the medical school, 1970–82

Peter A. Ward, MD, interim dean of the medical school, 1982–85

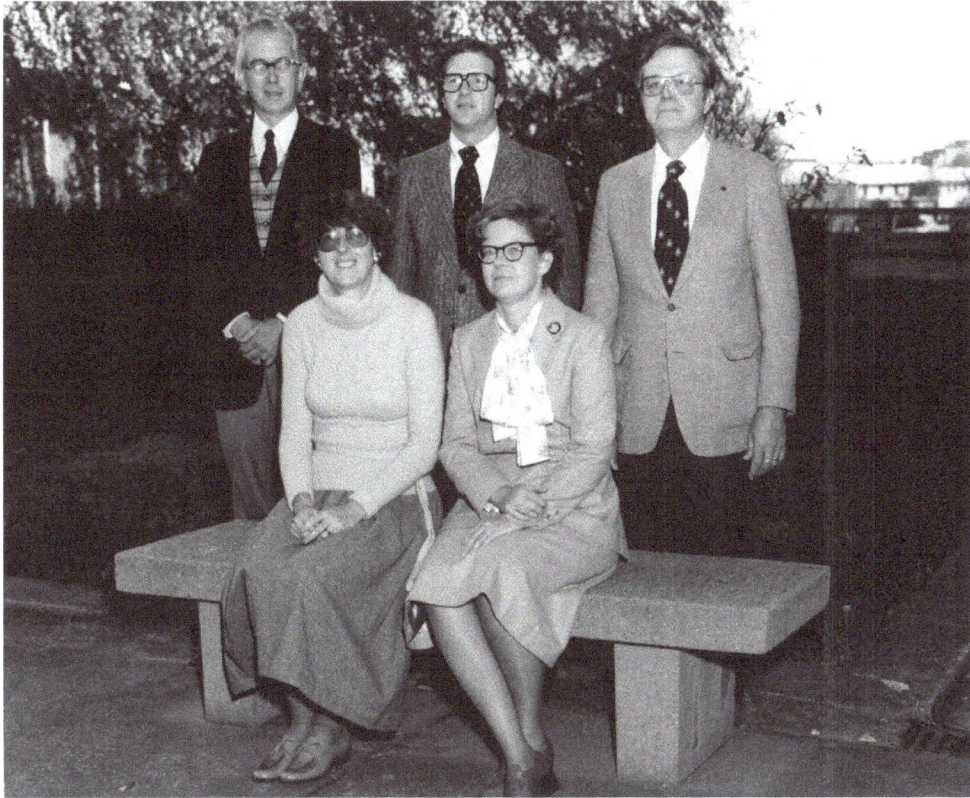

Figure 2.2. Original faculty. *Front row: S. Margaret Davies, MD; Shirley A. McCormick, MD. Back row: Terence C. Davies, MD; R. Dale Lefever, PhD; and Harry E. Schneiter, MD. Not pictured: James F. Peggs, MD*

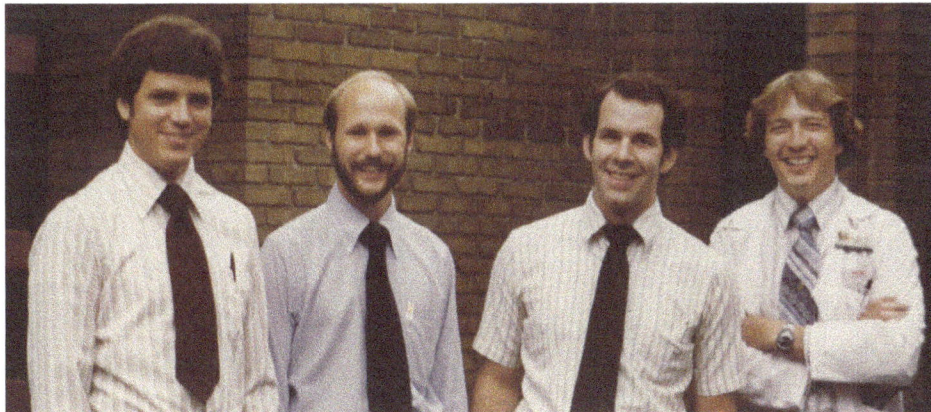

From left to right: Drs. O'Brien, Kearney, Frank, and Van Alstine (circa 1979–80).

NAME: John M. O'Brien, MD; Patrick J. Kearney, MD; Scott H. Frank, MD; and Fred J.
   Van Alstine, MD

ROLE: First class of residents

BIO: Members of the 1979 UMMS class and of the 1982 University of Michigan Family Practice residency class

Location on March 1, 1978: Somewhere in southeastern Michigan on a third-year clerkship

In February 1979, provisional accreditation for a three-year residency training program was received, and in July 1979, four recent UMMS graduates comprised the first class. The residency was reaccredited in 1982 and 1984 and has maintained full accreditation since then.

Once the accreditation application and the grant proposal were approved, the focus turned to getting arrangements finalized to have four new family practice residents rotate on services at the University of Michigan Hospitals.

Concurrent with the work being done on the residency accreditation and the training grant proposals, it was quickly becoming apparent that the clinical income being generated at the Chelsea Family Practice Center was not meeting the projections envisioned by the University based on the external report data that had been provided to the RPC during its deliberations. The department was more closely aligned with the hospital than the medical school, and the regular meetings between Drs. Davies and Lefever and representatives from hospital finance were often grim affairs. Ironically, in a foreshadowing of later developments of a more positive tone, many of those meetings took place in the conference room on the seventh floor of Medical Science I, the same room where resident conferences and clerkship teaching sessions would be held between 2013 and 2017.

In retrospect, it is easy to appreciate that the impetus for the University to establish the department was a forced marriage of sorts, imposed by the state legislature in exchange for funding for the replacement hospital, which opened as the new University Hospital in 1986. When the department did not meet the clinical projections based on the previous private practice model at Chelsea, there was not much tolerance for these budget concerns since the primary alliance for the department was with the hospital, not the medical school. Another issue was that several of the people who were supportive of the model of family practice and Dr. Davies were no longer with the University early in Dr. Davies's tenure as chair and later when some of the financial pressures escalated. Even before Dr. Davies arrived, Dr. Votaw left in 1977 to help start a new medical school at East Tennessee State University. Dr. Willson retired in 1978 as the chair of the Department of

---

"You Can't Make This Stuff Up"

In the early years of the department, which of these "common practices" were true statements?

The nurses wore hats.
Most of the physicians smoked cigarettes.
Fecal samples were mailed directly to the physicians in preaddressed envelopes.
Nurses wrote in red ink in the medical record.
Physicians wrote in black ink in the medical record.

All of these statements are true. As an additional teaching point, from that time up to the mid-1980s, no one could write in blue ink in the medical record because the photocopiers of that era did not make good copies of blue ink originals.

Obstetrics and Gynecology. Dean Gronvall left in 1982 for a position as an upper-level administrator in the United States Veterans Administration. Within the medical school and the institution, these three had been very strong advocates for the department as it was being established, and their absence left Dr. Davies without some allies that had been there in the build up to March 1, 1978.

Meanwhile, obstacles were encountered in establishing the process for placing family practice residents into the services of other clinical departments. It took a while to sort out some scheduling issues and determine the role of a family practice intern, which was a new model of resident training across the system. The department paid salaries for liaison faculty members from core clinical departments. These liaison faculty members, who were paid according to the number of months that family practice residents spent on services in those departments, played a key role in the early assimilation of family practice residents into other services. A major issue for faculty was a lack of understanding regarding the need for the four interns to leave their services each Wednesday afternoon to go to Chelsea for their continuity clinic. At that time, there was no model in other departments for their interns to leave their service to attend clinic, so it was a totally foreign concept to supervising residents and faculty physicians on other services to have the family practice interns leave the hospital on Wednesday afternoons to go to Chelsea to see their family practice patients.

Dr. Lefever served on behalf of Dr. Davies in the capacity of residency director and a conduit to the other departments for issues related to residency education. He took calls with the family practice interns to get a sense of the context and settings in which they were functioning. He coordinated resident recruitment and other functions associated with residency leadership in his role as director of educational development for the first five years of the residency.

In regard to medical student education, several proposals were submitted during this time frame requesting establishment of a required third-year family practice clerkship. None of these proposals was approved, but in the meantime, the department offered an outpatient elective based at the Chelsea Family Practice Center and in the offices of other community family physicians in the area.

Early on, the department became affiliated with the Integrated Premedical Medical (Inteflex) Program, which at that time was a combined six-year premedical and medical school degree program. A number of the residents in the early years of the residency program were Inteflex graduates, including two of the first four graduates.

In addition to the residency training grant funded in support of initial residency development, another early training grant was funded by the Division of Medicine, which supported medical student programs like preclinical preceptorships and student research assistantships. Even though there were no required clinical clerkships during this period, there were substantial teaching and course leadership activities within the Inteflex Program and in preclinical interviewing and other clinical skills experiences for all students.

Fun Fact: Did You Know?

Before computers and printers were invented, typewriters were used to create written documents like letters, memos, and grants. A highly coveted piece of equipment within the department in the early years, the IBM Selectric typewriter had the ability to backspace and make corrections without needing whiteout. The first computers that were used throughout the DFP were made by Televideo (no, that is not a typo) prior to the battle between Macintosh and IBM platforms for word processing supremacy.

Eventually an inpatient elective was offered at Chelsea Community Hospital along with the elective clerkship that was offered to students in the second half of their third year or in their fourth year.

In 1981, the central administrative offices moved from the second floor of Medical Science Building I to the Clinical Faculty Office Building (CFOB), which was also referred to as "the old interns' quarters," dating back to an earlier era when house officers stayed there overnight. CFOB was connected by tunnels to the old Main University Hospital and was adjacent to separate psychiatric hospitals. The Cancer Center now occupies most of this space. In 1984, the administrative offices were moved to 1018 Fuller Street, where most of the department's research faculty and staff are based to this date.

During the transition from CFOB to 1018 Fuller, the medical school conducted an external review of the department consistent with the routine process of reviewing department chairs on a regular basis. As noted, Dr. Gronvall had left to take a position in the Veterans Administration and was succeeded by an interim dean, Peter A. Ward, MD, who remained in that position for almost three years.

As alluded to in the list of July 1978 planning priorities, the development of a research program was an early goal. Dr. Davies made early connections to faculty at the School of Public Health, and he tried to establish some research linkages from his time at the Medical University of South Carolina. His initial choice for a director of research was unable to get approved for appointment by the medical school due to logistical issues. Subsequently, Charles B. Freer, MD, was selected to provide leadership for the research efforts, as reflected in the Research Task Force Report submitted by Dr. Freer and three other faculty members in June 1982. The challenges of adding research to the already heavy clinical and teaching loads of the faculty at that time are summarized among the conclusions of that report.

The committee felt that they were "perhaps on the threshold of a significant research effort" that would require research-oriented staff and general support. "We are confident," they said, that if "we can mobilize worthwhile research in the near future this will create the momentum for general enthusiasm and rapid expansion in this area of our work."[2]

While this report reflected the challenges of incorporating research into this new department, there was cause for great celebration later in June 1982 due to the graduation of the first four residency graduates. The event spanned two days, from June 17 to 18,

1982, and was held in the Rackham Auditorium. The presenters were a veritable who's who of family medicine. Among the audience members was also a UMMS graduate from the class of 1975 who would go on to become a member of the DFP faculty.

Later in June 1982, the first four graduates sent an open letter to members of the department. These four pioneers had taken a chance on this program before knowing if it would be accredited and used this letter to express their gratitude: "Three years ago four very different people made the same difficult decision. We elected not only to enter the infant specialty of Family Medicine but also to pursue this endeavor in the yet unborn Family Practice residency at The University of Michigan. We did not choose safety or stability, but rather the potential, and an air of excitement generated by the new faculty in the department. The three years since have combined unfilled promise and unpromised fulfilled."[3]

During an interview conducted in July 2015, Dr. Davies identified the graduation of those four residents as the most satisfying moment of his time as founding chair.[4] The rest of the open letter also described how the four graduates had established the Faculty Appreciation Senior Resident Award. This award continues to be bestowed yearly. (A list of recipients for this and other awards mentioned in the chapter is included in appendix C.)

The award is inscribed as follows: "To the faculty member who best typifies the principles of family medicine in character and in sensitivity to the residents' needs." In June 1982, the first recipient of this award, as determined by the senior residents in the first class, was R. Dale Lefever, PhD.

Three years later, the residents of the class of 1985 began the tradition of bestowing a second award at their graduation ceremony. The Resident Appreciation Award is displayed in the department administrative offices along with the Faculty Appreciation Senior Resident Award. This second award is "for encouragement and assistance beyond the call of duty." Across the years, its recipients have included office and clinical staff and faculty members. The first recipient was Betty K. Mull in 1985. Ms. Mull was an administrative assistant at the Chelsea Family Practice Center at that time and later was a residency coordinator based in the Ann Arbor administrative offices. This award continues to be bestowed yearly.

In 1986, another award was established and given to a graduating resident based upon a faculty vote. Lee A. Green, MD, was the first recipient of the Resident Teaching Award, which was given to him and subsequent recipients "in recognition of demonstrated interest, ability and commitment to family medicine education." Unlike other established awards, this was not given on an annual basis until 1998. In 2014, the Resident Teaching Award was renamed the Thomas L. Schwenk, MD, Resident Teaching Award in honor of Dr. Schwenk's many contributions to teaching and department leadership.

Following the review process in effect at the time, the department underwent a formal internal and external review beginning in 1983, five years after Dr. Davies's initial appointment. Due to significant financial concerns surrounding the department, the

Comments from "Building on a Vision" Document from 1998
Anniversary Celebration: The First External Review[5]

"In 1983, five years after the department was founded, the University conducted an external review to determine the viability of the department's future and the potential for the department to become a full participant in the institution. The review committee discovered a camaraderie and strength among our faculty, residents and staff members that demonstrated our devotion to family practice, to each other, to the department, and to the institution."

review process was initiated a year earlier than usual. Dr. Lefever chaired the internal review component process and submitted a report to the dean's office. Chairs from family practice departments at the University of Virginia and Medical College of Virginia were used as external consultants to the external review committee, which was chaired by George W. Morley, MD, a professor of obstetrics and gynecology.

From the perspective of those who were faculty members, residents, or staff members at the time, the process seemed to drag on forever, to the point that James F. Peggs, MD, a member of the internal review committee, wrote a letter to Dr. Morley in April 1984 regarding rumors in the community about the department's impending absorption into the Department of Internal Medicine as a "Division of Family Medicine." The lingering uncertainty of the fate of the department continued until the formal recommendations of the Family Practice External Review Committee were released in September 1984. The recommendations included a minority report proposing that the department be closed and that the existing combined internal medicine–pediatrics residency program be relocated in part to Chelsea. Even after the release of this report—which was positive in nature other than the minority report—there was no definitive action regarding the future status of the department. Given this uncertainty, Dr. Lefever wrote a letter to Interim Dean Ward in February 1985, requesting clarification of its status. The ultimate decision to maintain the department came months later in 1985, aided by decisions to use it as a key resource in developing a primary care referral network that would ultimately be called M-CARE.

Comments from "Building on a Vision" Document from 1998
Anniversary Celebration: The First External Review[6]

"The issue was whether they were going to continue us. A lot of us were very nervous about the whole thing."

R. Dale Lefever, PhD

"Our alignment was really with the University Hospital from 1978 to 1985. But when it was decided that we would stay, the University of Michigan's view was, 'If we're going to have a family practice department as part of the medical school, let's have it be one of the best in the country.'"

R. Dale Lefever, PhD

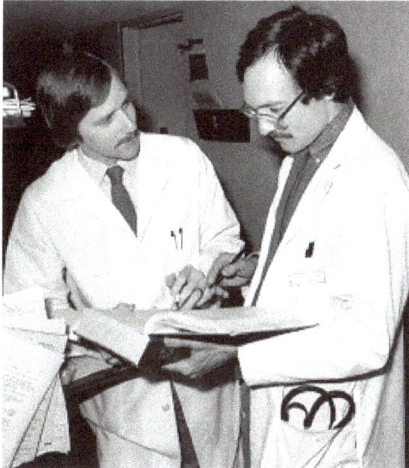

Figure 2.3. Dr. Peggs and Thomas C. Hupy, MD, UMMS class of 1982, residency class of 1985

As with the life span of most organizations, there are moments of chance that can lead to highly positive or negative outcomes. One moment of serendipity occurred when Patricia A. Warner, MPH, who was among the administrative staff, was assigned to work on the development of the M-CARE ambulatory care system. For a period of time, Ms. Warner and her staff were assigned office space in the 1018 Fuller building, which led to her greater appreciation of what family physicians could do in their roles in the health care system. At a time when few administrators within the medical center grasped the role family practice could play in the future of the health care delivery at the University of Michigan, she became a key ally in the coming years of the development of the department's clinical activities.

In a further linkage to the founding members of the department, Peggy Alford Campbell worked with Ms. Warner on the rollout of the new M-CARE Health Maintenance Organization and Preferred Provider Organization. Ms. Campbell continued to work for M-CARE and Ambulatory Care for a number of years, providing a connection back to 1978 and the first days of the department.

In the midst of all this uncertainty, Thomas L. Schwenk, MD, joined the faculty in September 1984 as assistant professor and director of graduate education. Dr. Schwenk was the 1975 UMMS graduate in the audience at Rackham two years earlier when the first group of residents graduated. He had attended the University of Utah for his residency training, then spent several years in community practice in Park City, Utah, before joining the faculty at the University of Utah Department of Family and Community Medicine. Upon returning to Ann Arbor, where he had received his undergraduate engineering and medical degrees, he served as residency director while Dr. Lefever transitioned into a role as the first assistant chair.

Along with Dr. Schwenk, several other faculty members who helped advance the research mission were hired from 1983 to 1985, including some support staff specifically devoted to research, as requested in the 1982 Research Task Force Report. Once it became clear that the University was fully committed to the department, new resources were secured and broader school-wide developments occurred to help address challenges. The traditional three-legged stool of patient care, teaching, and research was a complex issue to manage in a primary care–oriented department and in other clinical departments across the medical school. Among these school-wide changes, a major innovation that benefited the department from day one was the implementation of a clinical track option for faculty members.

As the calendar turned from 1985 to 1986, lots of changes were in the air, including the announcement that Dr. Davies was stepping down as chair and Dr. Schwenk would begin his appointment as interim chair on March 1, 1986, eight years to the day from when Dr. Davies began his term as chair. And in perhaps an even more ultimate moment of ironic timing, the new University Hospital opened in February 1986.

As reported in the spring 1986 issue of the Department of Family Practice Alumni Society Newsletter, the department was entering a new era. The newsletter also summarized the external review as follows in terms of departmental accomplishments:

1. The establishment of a full academic department from "scratch", placing the department's accomplishments in a particularly favorable light.
2. The high quality of the department's undergraduate and graduate teaching activities.
3. The high regard with which the residency program was held within the state and nation.
4. The extremely strong patient care operation developed at the Family Practice Center (FPC) at Chelsea.
5. The high quality of the community activities and community outreach programs.[8]

Joseph E. Johnson III, MD, began his term as dean of the medical school in 1985 and appointed Dr. Schwenk as the interim chair effective March 1, 1986. Dr. Johnson would be the dean for the next five years of the department's development as its scope expanded across clinical, educational, and research missions.

As the first eight years of the department came to a close, a new phase began under the leadership of Dr. Schwenk as he began his role as interim chair. Dr. Davies summarized

---

Comments from "Building on a Vision" Document from 1998 Anniversary Celebration: Terence C. Davies, MD[7]

"Dr. Davies spearheaded this team of truly competent, visionary, and—frankly—quite industrious brave individuals, and the Department of Family Practice, at least in my eyes, took on an academic flavor and intensity that were bound to lead to success."

Gary R. Gazella, MD

"Terry's vision and commitment were critical in those early difficult years, as was his unwavering belief that what he and the department were doing were absolutely important, not only for the department, but for the University of Michigan Health System."

Thomas L. Schwenk, MD

his eight years in the "Reflections" column in the spring 1986 issue of the Department of Family Practice Alumni Society Newsletter:

Harry Schneiter, Shirley McCormick, Jennifer Frank, Mike Liepman, Marshall Lyttle, Warren Garr, Charles Freer, Jim McGloin, Sarah Fox, Linda Cronenwett, Suzanne Heller, Jonathan Henry, John Severin . . . a roster of names that represent a historical commonality. Over the course of the past eight years, each of these individuals served on the full-time faculty of our department. They, the residents who have graduated and previous staff members must be counted with the faculty, residents, and staff of today for what has been done in the name of Family Practice at the University of Michigan.

As I reflect upon what has been achieved, it is images of people and personalities that predominate. Family Practice originated as a return to caring about patients as people; its greatest strength will always come from the fact that it depends upon caring and a commitment to humanistic values for its present existence and future survival.

These years at the University of Michigan have provided me with a full range of human emotions. I would never again wish to feel as lonely as I did in March of 1978; but I doubt that I will ever experience greater professional satisfaction than I did four years later, when the first residents graduated from the program. Since then there has been anxiety, uncertainty and frequent frustration; not infrequently it seemed impossible that the "new" primary care discipline of family practice could have a long-term future at this venerable but highly traditional institution. At all times the compensations have been the fellowship, the growing family of resident graduates and the conviction that we could match the excellence that the University of Michigan requires.

The first phase of program development might be descriptively titled the "period of endurance". While matters are in their formative phase they are also most vulnerable. Much has to be tolerated for the sake of survival. The emphasis has to be on quality rather than quantity, and most achievements occur in response to unexpected opportunities. The second phase occurs when the program begins to become indispensable to its supporting institution.

I am now completely confident that we have entered the second phase.

"A solid base has been established, and the department is now poised to grow, flourish, and take its place as a full peer among the clinical departments of the School."

Those last words are set in quotations because they are not mine but rather a statement made to me by Dean Johnson in a recent letter. I therefore regard it to be an enviable privilege that I can now relinquish my administrative role and recommit myself to the primary functions of an academician; and I have the enormous good fortune of recognizing a personal friend who is also a highly talented colleague as my successor, Dr. Tom Schwenk.[9]

The first eight years of the department were marked by a wide range of highlights and temporary setbacks. Dr. Davies established the foundation of an academic department of

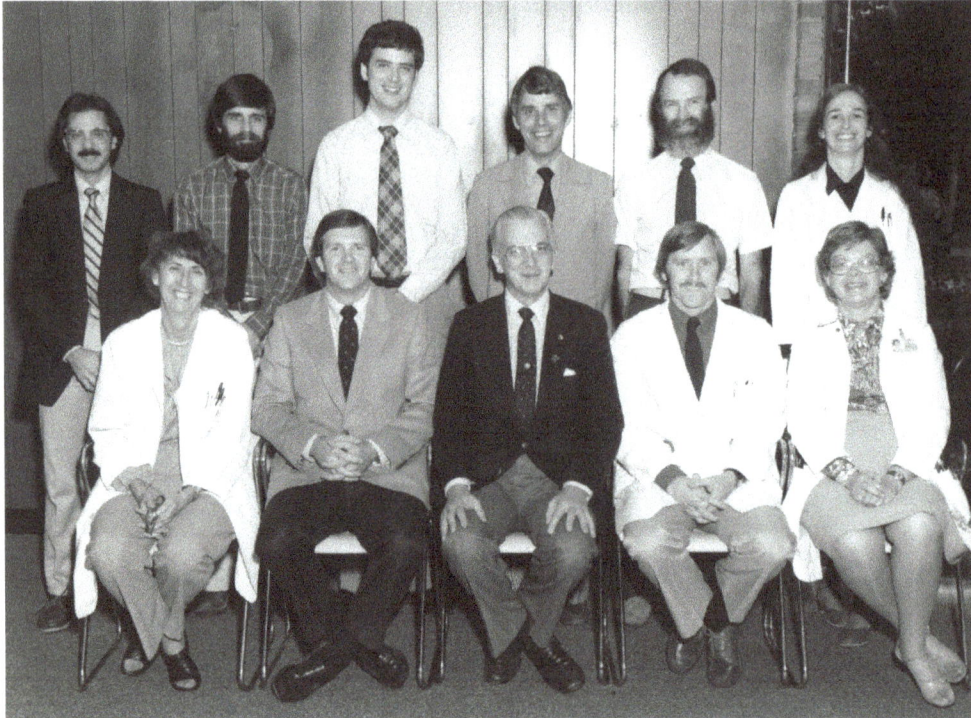

Figure 2.4. Group shot of faculty, 1982–83

family practice within an environment that was not always welcoming or appreciative of the strengths of this new specialty. The process and outcome of the internal and external reviews reinforced the need to build on this foundation by connecting the department more clearly to the medical school rather than the hospital. Dr. Schwenk brought his familiarity with the local environment as a UMMS graduate and his broader clinical and academic experience at the University of Utah to his role as interim chair, making him well positioned to lead the department in the next phase of its development.

Chapter 2 Timeline: Key Events/Individuals between 1978 and 1986

March 1, 1978	First day of the department
1978	First residency director appointed: R. Dale Lefever, PhD
1978	First service chief: Dr. Davies
1979	Accreditation and residency training grant is approved
July 1979	Entry of first class of four residents
1981	Move to Clinical Faculty Office Building
June 17–18, 1982	Family in Family Medicine Symposium
June 30, 1982	Graduation of first four residents
1983	First assistant chair: Dr. Lefever

1983 to 1984	Internal review process
1984	Move to 1018 Fuller
September 1984	Thomas L. Schwenk, MD, joins faculty
1984	Second residency director: Dr. Schwenk
1984–85	External review process
1985	First newsletter edition
March 1, 1986	Dr. Schwenk begins term as interim chair

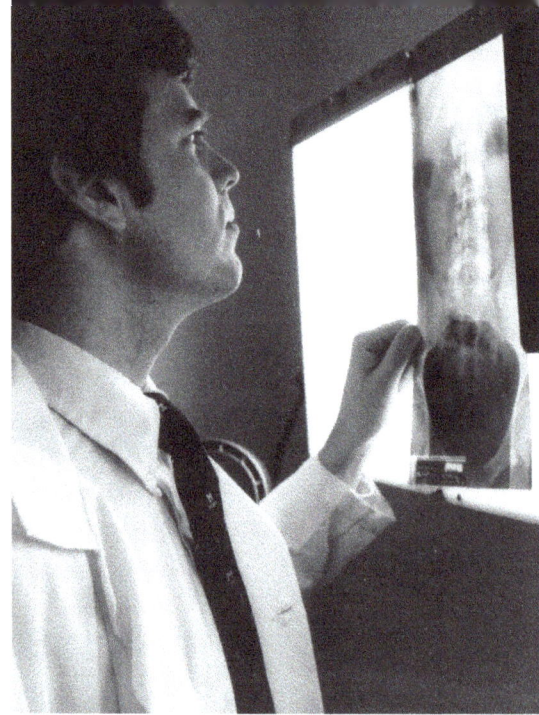
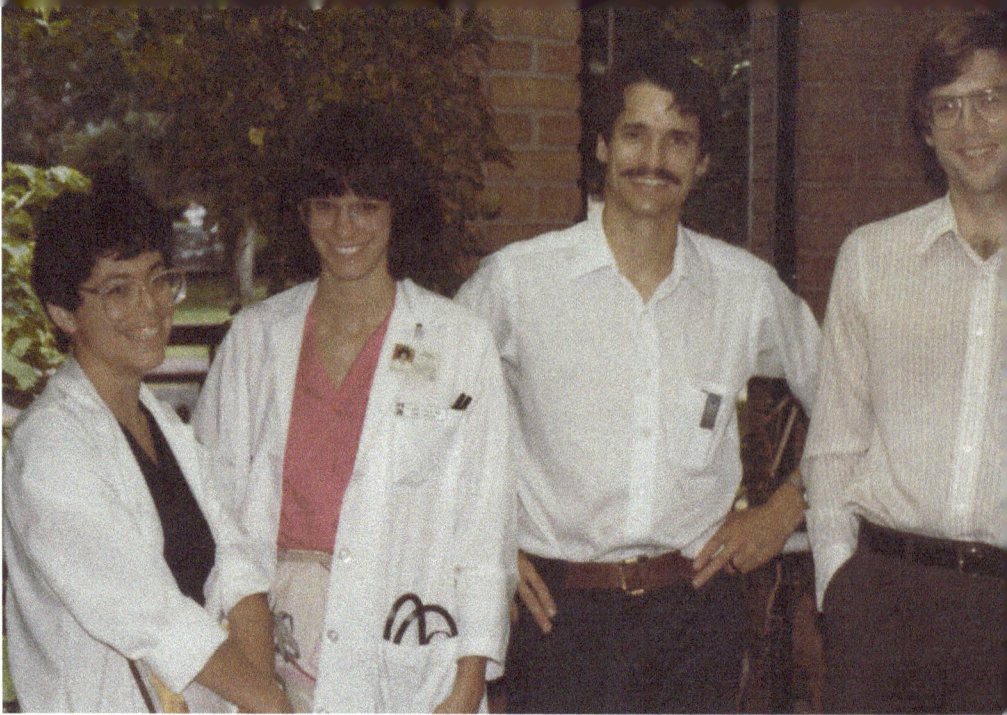

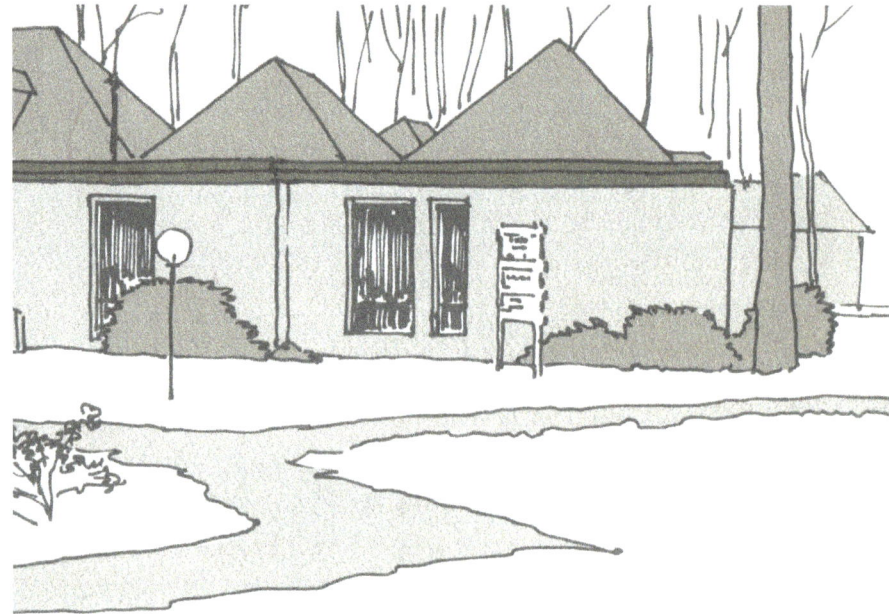

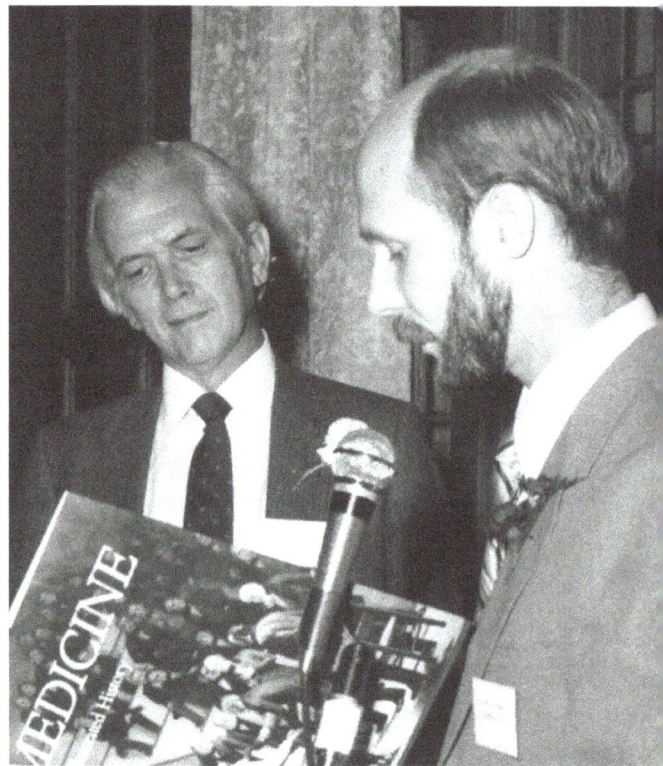

The University of Michigan

Department of Family Practice

Residency Program

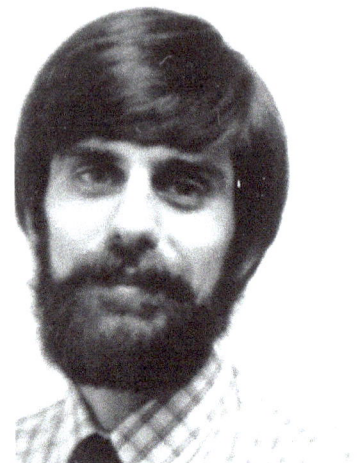
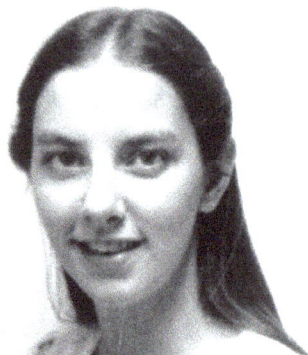
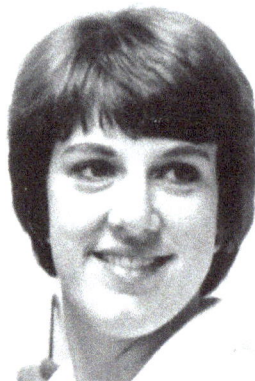
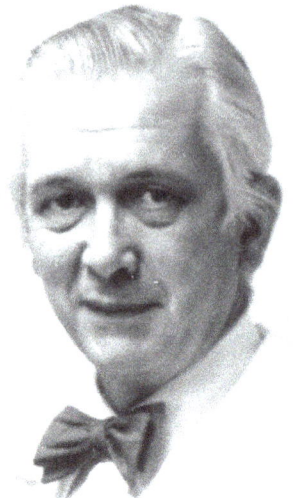

3

1986 to 1996

Getting More Connected to the
Academic Medical Center and
Expansion of Core Missions

The year 1986 marked a time of transition in leadership of the Department of Family Practice (DFP). Dr. Schwenk's first annual report as interim chair for 1985 to 1986 signaled the transition that occurred during that year and foreshadowed what was to come in the next decade. Dr. Schwenk acknowledged the foundation that was laid during the previous eight years and the opportunities that would arise in the coming years.

This is the first Annual Report to be published since the comprehensive department review was released in early 1986 (based on a review process extending over 1984–86) and the first report since the change in departmental leadership occurring on March 1, 1986. The past year cannot be described as one of boredom or lack of change. However, it also cannot be described as a year of great tragedy or adversity. Rather, the department made a transition from a period of foundation and early growth to one of great promise for strength and maturity. The transition was made with calmness, stability and confidence. This successful transition was due, in large part, to the vision of the department's founding chairman, Terence C. Davies, M.D., and to the maturity and optimism of its faculty.

The coming era in academic medical centers is characterized by several powerful forces, all of which bode well for primary care in general, and family practice in particular. The department will face the stress of choosing among too many opportunities, rather than too few, and the difficulty of managing growth, rather than retrenchment. This process has already begun, with the opening of the M-CARE Health Center at Briarwood, the pursuit of new external research grant support, the recruitment of new clinical and research faculty and the development of new educational and clinical initiatives based in the Medical School and University Hospitals. This 1985–86 Annual Report reflects a Department of Family Practice with outstanding potential already partially fulfilled. [1]

This phase in the history of the department includes many firsts, as the size and scope of the department continued to expand following the final resolution of the external review. Highlighting this evolution, the department developed closer ties to the medical school than in its first eight years.

Soon to become an annual event, the first State of the Department Address (SODA) was conducted by Dr. Schwenk in October 1986, seven months after his appointment as interim chair. All the employees of the department—faculty, residents, and staff—were assembled for an update on the current status of the department. This tradition continues to this day, with department employees from two administrative sites and six clinical sites suspending normal activities on a Wednesday morning to assemble for breakfast and an update on the departmental affairs. In more recent years, recipients of employee of the year awards have also been announced at SODA, with staff and faculty retreats following the meeting's completion. The location has changed several times due to the size of the group and finally settled at Weber's Inn on the west side of Ann Arbor, for both its capacity to handle the number of people and its relative ease of access from the widespread geographic locations of department sites.

A number of the firsts in this period were related to the clinical mission of the department. The Briarwood site opened in December 1986 on the south side of Ann Arbor, adjacent to the large Briarwood Mall, establishing the first clinical site in addition to the original location at Chelsea. Its location in Ann Arbor had great symbolic and tangible financial implications for the department.

In 1987 and 1988, Dr. Schwenk and others worked with faculty in the Department of Pediatrics and Communicable Diseases to formalize privileges for the care of newborn patients and delineation of pediatric admitting privileges for family practice faculty members. These concurrent developments in the outpatient and inpatient settings in Ann Arbor signaled the gradual integration of the department and its faculty and residents within both the academic medical center and the Ann Arbor community at large.

The opening of the Briarwood site was characterized by a combination of highs and lows, as is often the case with complex organizations or small businesses. One struggle was fighting the preconceived notion that family medicine would never work in Ann Arbor. The general sentiments of those outside the department were that "the patients are too sophisticated for family medicine. It will work in Chelsea and other rural communities, but not here." As a result, the original size of the Briarwood site was cut in half during the planning process, creating frustration among those who then were forced to work out of trailers when the demand for patient care quickly exceeded the projections for the smaller facility.

While there was great satisfaction in the fact that the department got the opportunity to demonstrate that its model of primary care would work in a large university town, the lack of appreciation for what the department and the specialty were capable of was disappointing. Eventually, a new larger practice site was built a short distance away in the Briarwood complex, but the sentiments about Ann Arbor's suitability for family medicine continued to create the impression that leadership at the University might never appreciate what the department had to offer in terms of clinical care, research, and education.

In February 1987, the formal process for identifying a new chair was initiated under Dean Johnson. At the end of June 1987, a search committee chaired by John Wesley, MD, an associate professor of surgery, submitted its report to the dean.

> The University recently reaffirmed its commitment to maintain a Department of Family Practice. The committee is convinced that an academically sound, high quality department is an achievable and desirable objective. The Medical Center is increasingly aware of the importance of primary care to its mission and image, and the Department of Family Practice can make a major contribution in this area. Success will, however, require institutional leadership and support. As the External Review Report of 1984 points out, it was difficult for the department to thrive when the institution's attitude about its very existence was ambivalent. The committee strongly believes that we now have an opportunity to attract an academically-oriented, forward-looking chairman. An assessment of the qualities we should be seeking in a chairman, as well as what will be required to attract such an individual, follows.[2]

After three full pages detailing key aspects of department strengths and weaknesses, the following conclusion provided a blueprint for moving forward once a new chair was appointed:

> The committee believes that the opportunity exists to recruit an academic leader to chair the Department of Family Practice, if the institution takes the necessary steps to let the department succeed. Critical issues include: an appreciation of the primary care mission of the department, acceptance of the department as a full member of the University community, and a realistic base of support for the department's activities. The committee believes that since we are committed to a Department of Family Practice, we should strive for a leadership position, including a research program based in primary care and a role in the training of academic leaders.[3]

Dr. Schwenk, the interim chair, and four other candidates for the position were identified by the search committee, and after the interview process and negotiations were

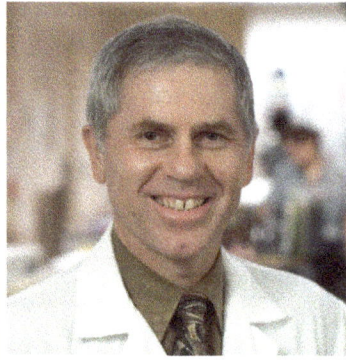

NAME: Thomas L. Schwenk, MD

ROLE: Second chair of DFP and first George A. Dean, MD, chair

BIO: Previously at University of Utah; 1975 UMMS graduate

Location on March 1, 1978: Salt Lake City, Utah, on a third-year family medicine resident rotation

completed, Dr. Schwenk was offered and accepted the opportunity to become the second chair of the DFP, effective September 1, 1988.

Concurrently with the chair search in 1987, while attending a medical school awards event, Dr. Schwenk and Kent J. Sheets, PhD, conceived of the notion of initiating an award to be given to a graduating student in honor of Dr. Davies. This award came to fruition in 1988.

As 1988 approached, the decision was made to celebrate the first ten years of the department with a series of formal events. Dr. Davies had stayed on the faculty following his resignation as chair, and he and Dr. Sheets worked with Dr. Schwenk and others to celebrate this occasion. The motto "Decade of Caring" was chosen to promote the series of events. Members of the Residency Planning Committee (RPC) and others who were integral to the founding of the department in 1978 were invited to an evening event in a private dining room within the University Hospital to kick off the series of celebrations. A series of events was linked to resident graduation and special anniversary events for faculty, residents, and staff throughout 1988.

One of the speakers at the Decade of Caring event at the University Hospital was Joseph V. Fisher, MD. Dr. Fisher was a UMMS graduate of the class of 1940 who had practiced in Chelsea for a number of years after serving in World War II and had been heavily involved in the efforts in the 1960s and early 1970s to lobby the University to start a department. He was president of the Michigan Academy of Family Physicians (MAFP) in 1971–72 prior to taking a faculty position at the Medical University of South Carolina, where he met Dr. Davies. During his comments at the Decade of Caring event, he detailed many of the activities of the local area family physicians and MAFP leadership to help nurture interest in family medicine among the UMMS students of that era, many of whom went on to leadership positions later in their careers.

Dr. Fisher closed his comments with these statements about Dr. Davies and the department: "I would be remiss if I failed to pay due honor to Doctor Terry Davies, your first chairman. The role of the pioneer is rarely an easy one, more often it is an arduous and at times a downright painful task. I have personal knowledge that a medical school rarely welcomes a new academic department among its firmly established disciplines and that is understandable. . . . Congratulations! And best wishes for many more productive years."[4]

In June 1988, Lisa J. Pierce was the first recipient of the Terence C. Davies, MD, Award. (A list of the recipients of this award through 2017 is included in appendix D.)

The Terence C. Davies, M.D. Award, named in honor of the founding Chair of the Department of Family Medicine, is presented annually to a graduating senior or seniors for clinical and scholarly excellence in family medicine. These students exemplify the qualities of the outstanding family physician: dedication to patient needs, intellectual curiosity, personal integrity, community service, and leadership.

Dr. Davies and his wife, Dr. Margaret Davies, were members of the faculty from 1978 to 1990. They played major roles in the Ann Arbor and Chelsea communities, were active teachers and course directors in the Inteflex Program, and Dr. Margaret Davies served on the Medical School Admissions Committee for many years. The Davies reside in Virginia near their three daughters.

Beyond the importance of honoring Dr. Davies, there was great symbolism since this award marked the first time that the name of the department and a specific faculty member and student were included in the official UMMS commencement program.

Following a rare vote of the faculty, the residency began to require resident research, mandating that each resident complete and present a research project as a requirement for graduation. After a series of efforts to mandate resident research projects with varying levels of success, the faculty came up with a compromise that resulted in broadening the definition of research into "original projects," which could be accomplished using a variety of approved methods and scholarly approaches. A faculty vote was used to determine the recipient following presentations made to the department, and in 1992, the first Resident Original Project Award was given to Robert B. Kiningham, MD. (A list of recipients of this award and others mentioned in the chapter is included in appendix C.)

The award is inscribed as follows: "In recognition of demonstrated interest, ability, and commitment to family medicine scholarship." In 2017, this award was renamed

Quote from the Recipient of the
2016 Terence C. Davies, MD, Award, Julie A. Blaszczak

"I am so humbled and honored to be chosen as the recipient of an award that represents such a remarkable and inspirational figure in family medicine. It is even more special to be joining the department he helped to create, alongside his wife as founding chair almost 38 years ago, and I can only hope to become the kind of physician he envisioned joining the department. This recognition will serve as motivation to continue to care fiercely for my patients."[5]

> ### Requiring All Residents to Complete an Original Research Project
> Rarely in the history of the DFP has a faculty vote ever been taken. In one of the few instances, a vote was taken regarding whether all residents should be required to do a research project. The tally of the votes is long lost, and most of the people who cast votes likely have forgotten how they voted, but the results of this faculty vote live on in the original project that is required of all third-year residents in order to graduate.

the Mack T. Ruffin IV, MD, Resident Original Project Award. For a number of years, fellows and residents have also been eligible to cast votes for the recipient(s) of this award in addition to the faculty.

Following Dr. Schwenk's appointment as chair in 1988, many developments and "firsts" continued to take place in the department's administrative, clinical, educational, and research components. The University Family Practice (UFP) service, which combined obstetrical and newborn care, was initiated in 1988–89. That same year, the first family physician fellow, David R. Mehr, MD, MS, completed the University's geriatric medicine fellowship administered by the Department of Internal Medicine. Dr. Mehr stayed on as a faculty member for several years following his fellowship, establishing research and academic connections between the DFP and the Division of Geriatrics in the Department of Internal Medicine that continue to this day.

Several years later, the sports medicine fellowship was initiated—the first DFP-administered fellowship. Dr. Kiningham was the first fellow to complete the sports medicine program in 1993 and later served as the second fellowship director following Dr. Schwenk's term.

In 1990, after twelve years with the department, Dr. Davies accepted an offer to become professor and chair of family and community medicine at Eastern Virginia Medical School. After Dr. Schwenk was appointed interim chair in 1986, Dr. Davies had stayed involved in activities across all department missions, including accepting a leadership role in medical student programs, particularly in the Inteflex Program, where he had been involved since 1978. He and his wife, S. Margaret Davies, MD, had been integral members of the department and the greater Chelsea and Ann Arbor communities as faculty members since 1978. Their three daughters grew up in Ann Arbor, and the eldest one, Nicola J. Davies, MD, followed her parents into family medicine. When she graduated from UMMS in 1992, she received the Terence C. Davies, MD, Award.

Also in 1990, Francine M. Bomar was hired as the first full-time clinical department administrator, reflecting the increasing size and complexity of the department across missions. The department's outpatient clinical base was expanded at the health system level under the auspices of the M-CARE administration, which oversaw development of several health maintenance organization and preferred provider organization models involving the department during this era. Individual family physician faculty members were incorporated into multispecialty M-CARE satellite sites in Northville and Plymouth

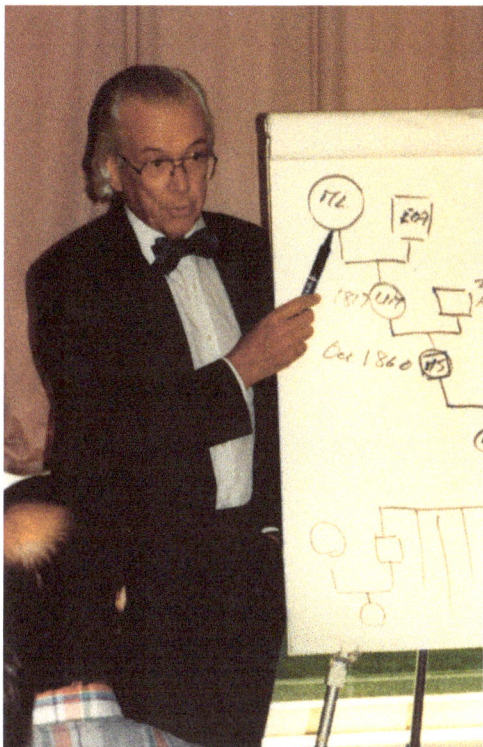

Figure 3.1. Terence C. Davies, MD

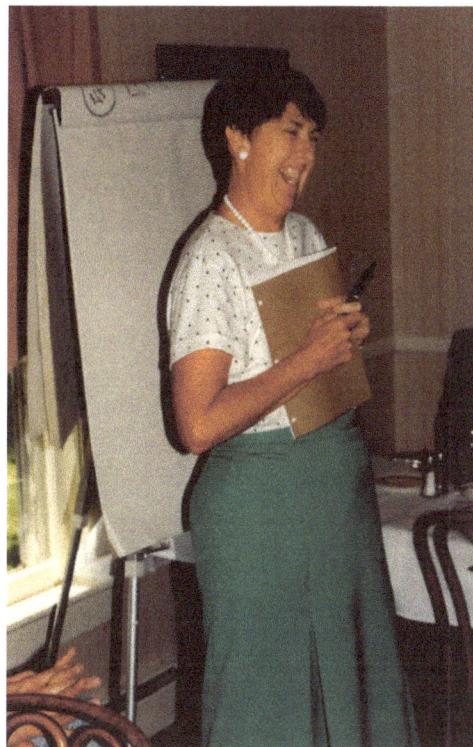

Figure 3.2. S. Margaret Davies, MD

in 1992 and eventually into one in northeastern Ann Arbor in 1993. None of these sites had a specific "label" as a family medicine center at that time like the one in use at Chelsea and Briarwood.

Meanwhile, the medical center began to purchase existing primary care practices in the county. In earlier stages of the department, several opportunities for merger or purchase of local practices had been considered but not completed. In 1993, the Ypsilanti practice of William P. Edmunds, MD, and Robert J. Fisher, MD, was purchased. Over a period of time, department faculty and staff were incorporated into the site, and eventually residents were assigned to that practice, making it a second training site for the residency program. It was also the first clinical site where the model of practice would be under the full responsibility of the department. At that time, both the Chelsea and Briarwood sites were still being administered in cooperation with the University Hospital. This new site was a major development in helping establish more autonomy in clinical operations.

Another significant event took place in 1993, as the department's relationship with the Corner Health Center in Ypsilanti became more formalized after more than ten years of department volunteer service. The Corner became a site for care of adolescent patients and children and continues to present day as a key component of teaching programs for fourth-year medical students and residents.

More consolidation of M-CARE satellite sites continued, and by 1994, there was a cadre of family physician faculty, including some who had previously been at the

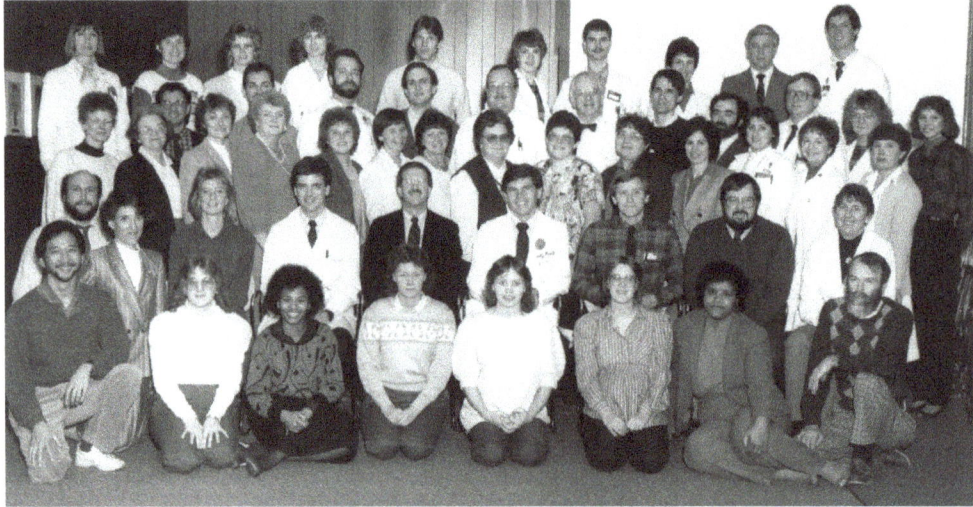

Figure 3.3. Group shot of faculty, residents, and staff, 1986–87

Plymouth and Northville locations, at a site on the northeast side of Ann Arbor on Green Road. Dr. Kiningham served as the medical director of this initial consolidation of family physicians into an integrated clinical setting in that part of town.

In 1996, the University opened a large new multispecialty site, the East Ann Arbor Health Center, at the corner of Plymouth Road and US 23. A family practice module was established there. The cohort of family physician faculty at the Green Road location, along with faculty from other sites, moved into the center to staff the larger clinical space. The Japanese Family Health Program had been established at the Green Road location in 1995, and it also moved to the new location. In 2006, the family medicine faculty and staff moved across Plymouth Road into its current location and was renamed Family Medicine at Domino's Farms.

As the department spread to the east from Chelsea into Ann Arbor and Ypsilanti, there was a need for more centralized meeting and educational space, especially as the department outgrew the available space in Chelsea. Space was rented off campus for a while at the Environmental Research Institute of Michigan (ERIM) before moving to the new East Ann Arbor Health Center when it opened in 1996.

On the heels of consolidating several faculty members at the Green Road site in 1994, a new Chelsea site was built in conjunction with Chelsea Community Hospital, opening in 1995. As more residents were assigned to the Ypsilanti site, a new building was built and opened in 1996 in conjunction with Oakwood Healthcare System and adjacent to Beyer Community Hospital, which had a long tradition of serving Ypsilanti and the eastern reaches of Washtenaw County. Finally, Dexter Village Family Physicians, a community practice in Dexter that had long been used as a clerkship teaching site, was purchased, and those physicians and staff became part of the DFP.

Though the UFP service was initiated in 1988–89 and privileges were developed in a similar time frame regarding care of newborns and admitting pediatric patients, working out collaborations in obstetrics took a while longer. In September 1994, the Family Practice Obstetrical Consultation and Privileges Guidelines were approved by all the necessary groups in both departments, accelerating the inclusion of family physicians in labor and delivery in the academic setting.

Concurrent with all this clinical expansion, there was finally progress within the medical school toward the long-standing goal of providing a required family practice clerkship to all third-year (M3) UMMS students. Some medical school leaders were concerned by the lack of ambulatory and primary care education for students as an accreditation site visit loomed, creating interest on the part of the dean's office to incorporate a required family practice clerkship into the third-year curriculum, replacing what previously had been an elective. The required M3 clerkship began in July 1996 and will be a major focus of the next chapter.

Much like the lack of appreciation of the potential for clinical family practice in Ann Arbor, a similar notion suggested that some of the department's educational efforts were unfit to be required of all UMMS students. While the following comment does not specifically speak to the inherent quality of education afforded to family practice residents and students participating in family practice electives at that point in time, it does show that the medical students who completed family practice electives paid attention to what was being role modeled by their family physician preceptors: "You guys and the pediatricians treat your students and your patients the nicest of anyone in the whole medical center."

Research development was another key focus within this period. Dr. Schwenk had taken advantage of strong support and recommendations and resources that arose from the chair search to bring in a cadre of new research faculty to strengthen the department's research mission. The medical school's creation of a formal clinical faculty track also enabled the DFP to retain faculty who had been appointed on the traditional instructional (tenure) track and were not going to meet the high standards for promotion but had proven to be very critical to success in core missions in education and clinical care.

"You Can't Make This Stuff Up"

At some point in 1995, word got out around the state that it was likely that a required third-year family medicine clerkship would be added to the UMMS curriculum. One day, Dr. Sheets got a phone call from a clerkship director at another school in the state. The phone conversation went something like this:

Caller: Hey, Kent, Tom Schwenk was talking at an MAFP meeting the other day about how you guys might be getting a required clerkship soon. Is that true?
Sheets: Yes, that is true.
Caller: One more question. Are you going to pay your community preceptors?
Sheets: Are you kidding? We don't have money to do anything like that.
Caller: Great. Thanks and good luck.

Some of these faculty members were also able to contribute to the research mission as the department evolved over the coming years.

In an effort to respond to the growth across missions, Dr. Schwenk announced plans for a sweeping reorganization of the department administrative structure in 1995. Previously, Dr. Lefever had been the only assistant chair since early in Dr. Davies's term as chair. Other than having faculty assigned to roles as residency director, medical director, and research director or chair of the research committee, there had not been much differentiation in terms of administrative structure at the upper levels of the department other than the existence of an executive committee that helped advise Dr. Schwenk on policies and procedures across missions.

After extensive review and consultation with individuals inside and outside the department, a new structure was established with assistant chairs assigned within the major areas of patient care, education, and research, along with a revised composition of the departmental executive committee. This reorganization was needed at the time and in retrospect also provided opportunities for more leadership experience for faculty who later became leaders within the department or elsewhere.

Dr. Lefever was given the specific title of assistant chair for planning and program development after his many years of service under the title of assistant chair, during which he had been involved in many aspects of new program development across missions. Barbara D. Reed, MD, MPH, was appointed the first assistant chair for research programs. James F. Peggs, MD, was appointed the first assistant chair for education programs and also was named the inaugural associate chair. Finally, Philip Zazove, MD, was appointed as the first assistant chair for clinical programs.

Concurrent with these changes, a new group was formed to focus on educational issues. The Education Steering Committee (ESC) was chaired by Dr. Peggs and consisted of Kent J. Sheets, PhD, as director of educational development; John M. O'Brien, MD, as residency director; Jennifer L. Hoock, MD, MPH, as assistant residency director for Ypsilanti; and Barbara S. Apgar, MD, MS, as assistant residency director for Chelsea.

The executive committee, composed of the chair and his administrative assistant, and the assistant chairs and other appointed members met monthly, as did the ESC. The composition and some of the position titles have changed over the years, but much of the original organizational framework is still in existence for both these groups.

To end this chapter, here are some of the notes from Dr. Schwenk's SODA from December 4, 1991. At the midpoint of this department phase of extensive growth, his comments recognized what had happened in the first five years of his leadership and envisioned what was to come over the next five years and beyond. Under the heading of "Stages of Department Growth and Success," he shared the following:

> Where does all this success get us? What's the point? The point is to assume a position of
> institutional leadership for sake of stability and strength, ability to influence entire system

with a set of values and principles we hold dear, we have to become more involved and influential in order to retain our relative independence; we need to reach out in order to set our own objectives; we have to continue to grow and change in order to be able to do things we always have done.

Some want to stay the way we are, return to earlier days. They don't believe we can stay the same, don't believe we want to change.[6]

What made Dr. Schwenk so sure in 1985 or 1986 that a "good family physician would always be successful"? In a January 2016 email, Dr. Schwenk said, "My personal experience to that point is that the power of what family physicians do, transcends politics and specialty bias and rivalries. All we had to do was get the opportunity to build a practice and we would prove ourselves. All this was based on my personal experience, and what I had seen in other places. What family physicians do is just intrinsically desired and valuable."[7] The department had been given the opportunity to demonstrate its academic capabilities following an external review and had responded.

Chapter 3 Timeline: Key Events/Individuals between 1986 and 1996

October 1986	First SODA (State of Department Address)
1986	Third residency director: John M. O'Brien, MD
1986	Second service chief: Dr. Schwenk
December 1986	Opening of the first Briarwood site
April 1987	Newborn Privileges Document
March 1988	"Decade of Caring" celebration
May 1988	Delineation of pediatric admitting privileges
June 1988	First student award: Terence C. Davies, MD, award
1988–89	Initiation of University Family Practice (UFP) service
1988–89	First family physician geriatric fellow: David R. Mehr, MD, MS
September 1, 1988	Dr. Schwenk begins term as second chair
October 1989	First faculty retreat
September 1989	Philip Zazove, MD, joins faculty
September 1990	First full-time department administrator: Francine M. Bomar
1991	First associate chair: James F. Peggs, MD
1992	First sports medicine fellow: Robert B. Kiningham, MD, MA
1993	Purchase of Edmunds and Fisher practice in Ypsilanti
1994	Opening of Northeast Ann Arbor site on Green Road
1994	Family practice and obstetrics consultation and privileges guidelines

1995	Reorganization of department leadership structure
1995	First assistant chair of education: Dr. Peggs
1995	First assistant chair of research: Barbara D. Reed, MD, MSPH
1995	First assistant chair of clinical programs: Dr. Zazove
1995	Opening of new Chelsea Health Center
1995	Expansion of residency to Ypsilanti
1995	Establishment of the Japanese Family Health Program
1996	First clerkship director: Dr. Peggs
1996	Opening of Ypsilanti Health Center
1996	Purchase of Dexter Village Family Physicians
1996	Opening of East Ann Arbor Health Center site on Plymouth Road

4

1996 to 2001

Establishing Credentials

The implementation of the required third-year clerkship beginning in July 1996 was a major milestone in the department's efforts to be fully integrated into medical student teaching. Previous proposals for a required clerkship had been denied, which, in retrospect, was fortunate since the department was not yet well positioned to implement such a major required student program. Drs. Schwenk and Sheets had both been involved in school-wide task forces and committees related to teaching in the ambulatory setting and had worked on proposals for options for primary care clinical experiences. When it became clear in 1995 that the opportunity to conduct a required clerkship was going to finally exist, the department was ready to respond properly, especially given the recent expansion of departmental clinical sites within the county. A Clerkship Steering Group (CSG) was assembled, composed of Drs. Sheets and Peggs and two junior physician faculty members, a fellow and the clerkship coordinator. The CSG set about the task of developing the materials and processes needed to implement a four-week family practice clerkship beginning in July 1996.

Dating back to the early years when Drs. Davies and Lefever were successful in writing training grants to support residency and predoctoral program development, the Department of Family Practice (DFP) continued to be successful in gaining a number of other important grants, including a faculty development grant for faculty and preceptors in sites around the area and the state. Similar success with residency training grants had also continued for much of the previous phase as well.

The four-week clerkship was a success from the beginning, gaining the highest student ratings of any required clerkship from its initial offering in July 1996. In addition to using department sites, students were placed in the offices of local community family physicians, statewide community residency programs, and community family physician preceptor sites. Many community residency programs already affiliated with Wayne State or Michigan State were eager to finally get a chance to have contact with third-year University of Michigan Medical School (UMMS) students as a way to increase their pool of potential residency applicants.

As the clerkship was being implemented, the DFP went through another internal and external review. The chair search committee had done a more limited review in the process of doing their work in 1987–88, but this was the first in-depth review since 1984–85. The department's second review, conducted in 1996, included a comprehensive internal examination of the department's status and future needs in the areas of education, research, and clinical programs and external scrutiny by academic leaders from other family medicine departments.

The reviewers lauded the department's reputation as a top-ranked program with excellent faculty and particular strengths in research and scholarship, including strong extramural grant funding, and confirmed the importance of the required third-year clerkship as an essential component of the department's success.

Most notably, the review confirmed that the DFP and its reputation were more widely known and established nationally with other academic family medicine departments and colleagues than inside the UMMS. To promote wider internal visibility and more interaction, the review recommended that the department secure more central administrative, teaching, and research space within the medical center. The reviewers also suggested changing the department's name from the Department of Family Practice to the Department of Family Medicine (DFM) to reflect the department's academic orientation and national reputation. One of the reviewers was Elizabeth A. Burns, MD, MA, a professor and head of the Department of Family Medicine at the University of Illinois at Chicago College of Medicine and a member of the UMMS class of 1976.

A. Lorris Betz, MD, PhD, was the interim dean at the time immediately following the review, having replaced Giles G. Bole, MD, who had initiated and presided over the review process before stepping down. Interim Dean Betz sent a letter dated September 16, 1996, to Dr. Schwenk about the outcome of the review and the next steps in the process.

You and your faculty should be proud of your accomplishments since you were appointed Chair eight years ago. The department is nationally recognized as one of the top academic departments of family practice in the country. Your faculty have been successful in obtaining external research funding, the department has developed and initiated a required clerkship in family medicine, and you have assisted in the expansion of our clinical capabilities in primary care. Based upon national trends in health care, your discipline is expected to show substantial growth in the future and the Executive Committee recognizes the growing importance of your department in our Medical Center.

Nevertheless, it is clear that the department is not as well integrated into the Medical Center as it should be. The physical isolation probably contributes to this poor integration. However, the institution does not yet have a clear vision of the unique role of a department of family medicine in a tertiary academic medical center like ours. . . . I believe that we will have an opportunity to enhance the position of your department in the Medical Center, but this will require cooperation, collaboration, and the development of a positive attitude among your faculty. I ask that you submit to me a strategic plan to address the above issues. Once we reach agreement on this plan, I will work with you to better integrate the department physically within the Medical Center and I will explore the possibility of changing the name of your department to the Department of Family Medicine.[1]

Other key events took place following the external review. The new Briarwood site opened in February 1997, providing much needed additional space and a building devoted solely to department faculty and staff. The year 1997 also marked the introduction of a departmental educational relative value unit (RVU) system, which continues to be used twenty years later. After a series of attempts to develop a process for identifying core teaching activities to improve allocation of faculty work effort, the decision was made to incorporate a formal system based on formulas and faculty self-reports. The system would document faculty contributions to student and resident education, grand rounds presentations, and other core teaching activities on a quarterly basis. The department educational RVU system was based in part on similar systems at the medical school level and was administered by Dr. Lefever at the onset.

Several new assistant chairs were appointed in 1997. Dr. Green was appointed as the assistant chair of research, and Raymond R. Rion, MD, replaced Dr. Zazove as the assistant chair of clinical programs. Also in 1997, Dr. Zazove was appointed west region medical director within the Ambulatory Care Services of the University of Michigan Hospitals and Health System. This was the first significant appointment of a family physician faculty member to a leadership role within the clinical leadership structure of the institution.

A new site was opened in Livonia in 1997, spreading the footprint of the department's clinical efforts to the east and to the western edge of Wayne County. Three recent resident graduates were part of the core group of faculty that opened that site. Another new building was opened east of downtown Dexter in 1998, and the practice that had been purchased several years earlier moved to that site along with additional faculty and staff who were recruited to fill the larger space. Also in 1998, a new site was opened in Stockbridge, built in conjunction with Chelsea Community Hospital, which spread the footprint of the department to the west and into Livingston County. Two faculty physicians and a physician assistant were the initial clinicians at the Stockbridge Health Center.

Dr. Peggs gained recognition outside the department in March 1998. He was the recipient of the coveted Silver Shovel Award, bestowed upon him by a vote of members

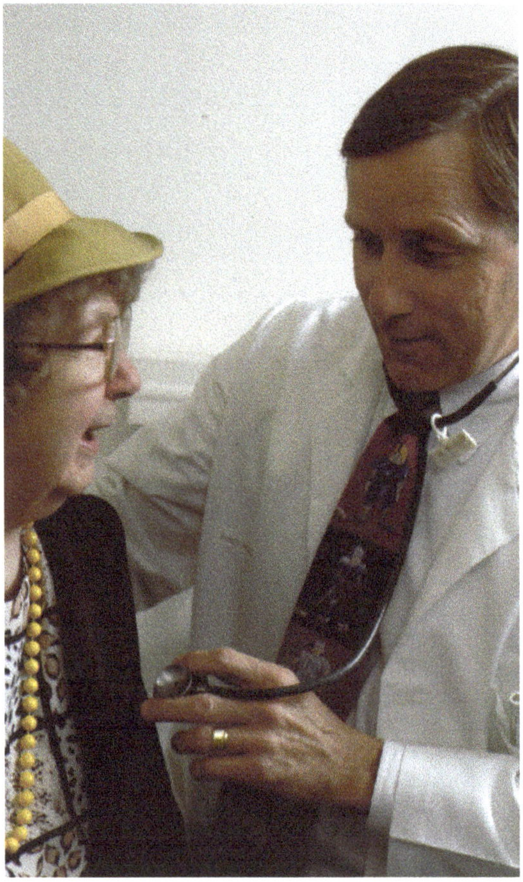

Figure 4.1. Dr. Peggs and a patient

of the Galens Medical Society, the longest existing student organization in the institution. His role and visibility as the first required clerkship director, along with his involvement in other student activities, led to this singular achievement in the history of the department. In 1999, he was also named the MAFP Family Medicine Educator of the Year, the first time that one of the faculty had received that honor.

In May 1998, the department marked its first twenty years with a celebration built around the theme of "Building on a Vision." Faculty, residents, staff, friends of the department, and graduates gathered for a series of presentations and a formal dinner. One segment of the celebration did its best to try to predict the future with a symposium titled "The Family Physician in 2008: What Should We Teach? How Should We Teach?"

Comments from "Building on a Vision" Document
from 1998 Anniversary Celebration

"Our relationship with Chelsea Community Hospital has been especially important to our success. The commitment to excellence shared by the hospital and our department have led to a beautiful new Family Practice Center on the Chelsea campus and in Dexter; as well as a new building and practice in Stockbridge."[2]

James F. Peggs, MD

In conjunction with the anniversary event, a large illustrated brochure featuring photos, quotes, and highlights of the first twenty years was developed and disseminated to alumni, current members of the department, and other friends. Among the unique features of this brochure was an insert listing the names of residency and fellowship graduates up to 1998, including their current practice locations. In addition to the large number of graduates who had stayed to practice in many communities throughout Michigan and even within the DFM, the number of states and countries where residents were in practice outside Michigan was impressive. At that point in time, the practice locations for resident and fellow graduates outside Michigan included Arizona, California, Colorado, the District of Columbia, Florida, Illinois, Indiana, Louisiana, Maryland, Massachusetts, Minnesota, New Hampshire, New Mexico, New York, North Carolina, Ohio, Oregon, Pennsylvania, Virginia, Washington, and Wisconsin, as well as China and Ontario.[3]

In June 1998, the residency reached the milestone of one hundred graduates. Starting with that first class of four graduates in 1982, the size of the entering classes had varied from six to eight across the intervening years, but the steady progression of residents completing the program, aided by the expansion to the second site in Ypsilanti several years earlier, facilitated the crossing of the milestone.

The original plans for the department and residency approved in 1976 called for ten residents in a class as early as 1980, but it was not until the entering class of 1997 that this goal was achieved. Currently, the class size is at eleven for the 2017–18 year with approval to recruit thirteen interns for the entering class of 2018–19.

In 1998, the residents initiated another award that continues to be bestowed on a faculty member at residency graduation each June. The Award for Excellence in Teaching is presented "in recognition of outstanding contributions to resident education." A. Evan Eyler, MD, was the first recipient in 1998.

As Dr. Schwenk noted in his "Reflections" column in the 1998 fall/winter alumni newsletter, "What we are really celebrating is an environment, a supportive scholarly atmosphere, a quest for excellence that respects a wide range of interest and methods, and

Progression of Cumulative Number of Residency Graduates	
1982	4
1990	50
1998	100
2003	150
2008	200
2014	250
2017	289
2018	300 (projected as of 10/1/2017)

Comments from "Building on a Vision" Document
from 1998 Anniversary Celebration

"Dr. Schwenk has always been kind enough to credit me with bringing a certain humanism to the department. But I think Dr. Schwenk has managed a more notable feat—continuing that humanism while adding an intellectual and academic level of achievement that I'm very proud of. His efforts have earned the department an academic status that is second to none."[5]

Terence C. Davies, MD

a tolerance for the many ways academic family physicians and department staff members contribute to the department's success."[4]

Another recommendation from the 1996 external review had been for the department to be more formally connected to and established within the medical center. This had meant moving a cadre of faculty and staff members out of 1018 Fuller. Other location options were considered, but finally space in Women's Hospital was secured and plans were made for moving administrative, educational, and research faculty and staff into space on the ground floor. Rather late in the process, half the space originally secured for the department administrative offices was taken away for use by other units in a similar fashion to the space reduction at the first Briarwood site. Thus, only a limited group of faculty and staff were able to move from 1018 Fuller to Women's Hospital. The chair, assistant chair, and residency director, along with their associated staff, moved to the new space in May 1999. Additional swing space was available for use by residents, faculty, and staff, as was a conference room that was used for clerkship and resident teaching conferences.

Department grand rounds, morbidity and mortality conference presentations, and faculty meetings were moved to the medical center, using the Ford Auditorium at the University Hospital for these major gatherings and educational programs. Resident conferences were held in the new space in Women's Hospital, as were most regular meetings of groups such as the Executive Committee and Education Steering Committee.

Prior to the move to Women's Hospital, a series of locations had been used outside the medical center once the size and complexity of the department outgrew the capacity of the Chelsea site and a more central meeting location was needed. While being unable to move more of the 1018 Fuller contingent to Women's Hospital was disappointing, it did mark a shift in the focus of department and residency leadership to the center of the action in the academic medical center, as had long been a departmental goal.

As many looked forward to the turn of the century amid concerns over what might happen to the world's computer infrastructure on the date of the cryptically named Y2K, the department worked to establish the Complementary and Alternative Medicine Research Center in 1999. This marked the beginning of a tradition of education, scholarship, research, and clinical care in complementary and alternative medicine, which is currently referred to as integrative medicine. The tradition and importance of incorporating integrative medicine across departmental missions continue to the present, nearly twenty years later.

In February 1999, a major transition took place in the department's inpatient clinical care operations when the University Family Medicine (UFM) service opened at the University Hospital, providing a second option for inpatient care and the training of family medicine residents and eventually fourth-year medical students. After twenty years of providing inpatient care at Chelsea Community Hospital, it was a significant development for department faculty and residents to begin to offer inpatient care in the heart of the medical center. William E. Chavey II, MD, a resident graduate who had returned as faculty after several years in practice in North Carolina, was the initial UFM service chief. There have been major adjustments and refinements in the years since 1999, but the UFM service continues to be a strength of the DFM's clinical and educational programs for residents and fourth-year medical students.

In 1999, the department also made its first appearance in the rankings of National Institutes of Health (NIH) grant funding of family medicine departments. The department was ranked third for that year.

One of the factors in establishing the second residency site in Ypsilanti had been the presence of Beyer Community Hospital. Beyer provided a second community hospital setting for care of patients from the Ypsilanti practice as well as another site for inpatient training for the residents. Beyer had experienced financial problems and was purchased by the Oakwood Hospital Healthcare System based in Dearborn in 1991, but the problems continued even after Oakwood partnered with the DFM to build the Ypsilanti Health Center, which was physically connected to Beyer and had opened in 1996. When it became obvious that Beyer was starting to fail as a reliable setting for inpatient care, the patients previously cared for at Beyer were admitted to UFM along with patients from other sites in the greater Ann Arbor area. Beyer Hospital closed in 2000 and eventually was purchased by a private corporation and converted to a bariatric care center.

Later in 2000, two of the department's outpatient sites also closed, the western and eastern sites in Stockbridge and Livonia, respectively. The medical center was undergoing some financial concerns that affected the department, and those sites were among the casualties of the retrenchment of a broader network of primary care sites in southeastern Michigan.

Within the research mission area, the Great Lakes Research Into Practice Network (GRIN) was founded in 2000. This statewide primary care research network, led by faculty from the DFM and the MSU Department of Family Medicine, combined office practices in family medicine, internal medicine, pediatrics, obstetrics and gynecology, and independent-practice nursing. Dr. Green served as the network's first director.

With this as a backdrop, the DFM went through another internal and external review in 2001. Once again, a major focus of the external review was on budgetary issues since the medical center was facing financial concerns, including repercussions of prior overexpansion of the outpatient network, which had already led to the closing of the Stockbridge and Livonia sites. The next internal and external review reports would set the stage for the next ten years of further development of the department. Now that the DFM had established itself on the national stage, over the next ten to fifteen years, the department began to focus on consolidating its gains and refining its priorities across its core missions of patient care, education, research, and service.

Chapter 4 Timeline: Key Events/Individuals between 1996 and 2001

July 1996	Beginning of M3 required clerkship
1996	Opening of Ypsilanti Health Center
1996	Second department review
1997	Department name is changed to Department of Family Medicine
February 1997	Move to second Briarwood site
1997	Initiation of educational relative value unit (RVU) system
1997	Opening of Livonia Health Center
1997	Second assistant chair of research: Lee A. Green, MD, MPH
1997	Second assistant chair of clinical programs: Raymond R. Rion, MD
May 1998	Twenty-year celebration event, "Building on a Vision"
1998	Opening of Dexter Health Center
1998	Hundredth resident graduates
1998	Opening of Stockbridge Health Center
1999	Establishment of Complementary and Alternative Medicine Research Center
February 1999	Establishment of University Family Medicine (UFM) inpatient service
May 1999	Move of administrative offices to Women's Hospital
1999	First National Institutes of Health (NIH) funding ranking among family medicine departments: third place
1999	Dr. Peggs is named MAFP Family Medicine Educator of the Year
January 2000	Closure of Beyer Hospital
2000	Closure of Stockbridge Health Center
2000	Closure of Livonia Health Center
2000	First University of Michigan Medical School female faculty member is promoted to rank of clinical professor: Barbara S. Apgar, MD, MS
2001	Third internal review process

5

2001 to 2011
Generating Support and Success
of Development Efforts

The internal and external reviews of the Department of Family Medicine (DFM) that took place in 2001 confirmed its growing reputation across missions at the institutional and national level. The two external reviewers—Alfred O. Berg, MD, MPH, from the University of Washington and Stephen P. Bogdewic, PhD, from Indiana University—identified a number of strengths across missions. These strengths included highly qualified faculty and staff, a highly respected chair, and outstanding educational programs. They also acknowledged recent accomplishments in research endeavors and ambulatory clinical activities. In particular, they noted that the department had achieved a national reputation based on its success across the areas of education, research, and clinical service.

Dean Allen S. Lichter sent Dr. Schwenk the full review and a letter summarizing the next steps in the process following the external review. After sharing the review and Dean Lichter's letter with key departmental leadership, Dr. Schwenk focused his response to the dean on issues related to developing a plan for research; reviewing support for education; continuing an active debate of the issue of properly supporting primary care sites, most notably the Ypsilanti Family Practice Center; exploring development as a source of recurring support; and reviewing general fund support. While not all of the proposals made to Dr. Lichter were fully enacted, enough of them were for the department to continue to prosper and thrive for the next ten years, including stabilizing support for the clinical enterprise after expanding to Livonia and Stockbridge and then having to close those sites after two to three years.

Several key outcomes were attributable to earlier investments in both people and technology, one of which resulted in the development and licensing of a prompt and reminder system named ClinfoTracker, which was designed as a platform for studying cognitive aspects of prompting clinicians in primary care settings. Dr. Green and Donald E. Nease Jr., MD, were key to developing this platform and incorporating it into clinical and research applications. Eventually ClinfoTracker was sold to a private company, which marketed and sold it as Cielo Clinic.

Several changes in key leadership positions took place during this time period. In 2002, Jean M. Malouin, MD, MPH, was named the third assistant chair for clinical programs, and Eric P. Skye, MD, was appointed as the fourth residency director, replacing Dr. O'Brien, who had served in that role for sixteen years, the longest stint in that key role to date. Dr. O'Brien was chosen as the MAFP Family Medicine Educator of the Year in 2005, and in 2007, Dr. Skye received that same award.

Several other faculty members received significant regional and national awards during this period. Dr. Schwenk was elected to the Institute of Medicine in 2002 and received the Society of Teachers of Family Medicine (STFM) Recognition Award in 2003. Also in 2003, Michael L. Szymanski, MD, was named the MAFP Family Physician of the Year, the first faculty member to receive that honor. In 2004, Dr. Ruffin was appointed the third assistant chair for research programs, replacing Dr. Green in that position. In 2006, Dr. Green was appointed as the initial assistant chair of information management and quality.

In response to institutional and national initiatives, the department made significant changes to the way family medicine was practiced and studied. The creation of the new position of assistant chair of information management and quality reflected the need to have additional leadership and expertise in support of these new efforts.

In 2004, the department began to transform the way care was delivered and to implement innovative components of care into its clinical programs. Efforts affected many aspects of care in the department's outpatient sites, such as patient access, patient care teams, management of paperwork and communication, population-based management, and integration of teaching and research into clinical care. The implementation of CareWeb (the health system's homegrown electronic medical record) and continuing development of ClinfoTracker also supported these efforts.

The efforts to redefine the process of care continued in 2006 as the Briarwood site piloted electronic visits, and across sites there were efforts to change appointment lengths to twenty minutes rather than the traditional fifteen- and thirty-minute time frames. Group visits were explored, and a longitudinal chronic illness management program using registered nurses was also pilot tested.

Finally, in 2011, efforts led by Dr. Malouin were key to the state of Michigan being chosen to participate in the Centers for Medicare and Medicaid Services' Multi-Payer

Advanced Primary Care Practice Demonstration project. Dr. Malouin led the state's project, the Michigan Primary Care Transformation Project.

One of the significant outcomes of the 2001 review was the recommendation that the department continue its evolution by adding a development officer, who would be partially funded by the medical school and the development office for a period of at least three years. Amy C. St. Amour was chosen to be the first person in this position beginning in 2003.

The success of another anniversary event held in 2004 to celebrate the first twenty-five years of the department provided evidence of the value of a more formal development focus. The timing was right for having someone specifically reach out to alumni and friends of the department to inform them of recent accomplishments and to establish policies and procedures for giving to support specific program missions. This era was notable for an explosion in the number of awards and scholarships awarded to medical students and residents, with most of the money that was awarded going toward reduction of debt for medical students who had matched into family medicine residency programs.

The first student scholarship, the Department of Family Medicine Senior Scholarship, was awarded in 2004. There were two inaugural recipients, Tracy T. Bozung and Andrew H. Heyman. This has been the only time when two recipients of this scholarship were chosen in the same year. (A complete list of recipients of this scholarship and others mentioned in the chapter is included in appendix D.) This scholarship is "awarded to a senior medical student based on academic achievement, performance in the family medicine clerkship, a demonstrated commitment to the principles of, and a career in, family medicine and demonstrated financial need."

In 2005, Katherine J. Gold, MD, MSW, MS, was the first recipient of the William Clippert Gorenflo Research Award in Family Medicine. This is the only current award that can be awarded to a medical student or a first- or second-year family medicine resident. Among the medical student recipients, several of them have been preclinical students, so this award is not limited to students who have already matched into family medicine. Dr. Gold was a resident at the time she received the award, and since that time, she has served as the faculty mentor to other recipients of this award. This award is "awarded to a medical student or resident who is doing research with a family medicine clinical or research faculty member. This unique award provides incentive and rewards passion and enthusiasm for research. The William Clippert Gorenflo Research Award was established by Daniel W. Gorenflo, PhD, a former research investigator in the Department of Family Medicine, in honor and memory of his father who died in 2004 at the age of 83."

In 2005, Sarah Vanston was the first recipient of the Harold Kessler, MD, Scholarship in Family Medicine. As with the Gorenflo Research Award, this scholarship is awarded before students have matched into a specialty, so not all the recipients have entered family medicine residency training following medical school. This scholarship "supports a senior medical student based on academic achievement during the first three years of medical school, performance in the family medicine clerkship, a demonstrated commitment to the principles of and a career in, family medicine, and demonstrated financial need, as well as, an interest and dedication in helping rural and/or medically underserved populations. The scholarship was established by Susan, Barbara and Sam Kessler in honor of their father who passed away in 2003."

In 2005, James F. Dolan was the inaugural recipient of the Kenneth and Judy Betz Family Medicine Scholarship. This scholarship is "awarded to a senior medical student based on academic achievement, performance in the family medicine clerkship, a demonstrated commitment to the principles of, and a career in, family medicine and demonstrated financial need. The Betzs, who reside in Grand Rapids, established this scholarship in recognition of their daughter's achievements in family medicine. Mrs. Betz passed away on June 24, 2017, at the age of 70, just three days shy of her 71st birthday. Yet, her legacy lives on in perpetuity through the Kenneth and Judy Betz Family Medicine Scholarship."

In addition to the increase in the number of scholarships awarded in May 2005, that year also marked the initiation of the Development Advisory Committee (DAC). The DAC was led by Ms. St. Amour and Dr. Lefever with additional involvement from Dr. Schwenk. Two of the DAC members from the beginning were representatives from the Residency Planning Committee (RPC), Gary R. Gazella, MD, and Dale L. Williams, MD. Other early members of the DAC were medical school or residency program graduates who had stayed in contact with the department in various fashions. Before the formation of the DAC, the department began to sponsor a family medicine reception in conjunction with the annual fall event hosted by the Medical Center Alumni Center (MCAS), which was held on a home football game weekend. The family medicine reception was generally held on Friday afternoon in between larger general interest sessions in the MCAS schedule, creating a chance for personal connections to be developed between the department and family physician medical school graduates.

The department had made previous attempts to participate in MCAS events, but the addition of a development officer and a formal committee provided greater structure and purpose. In this same time frame, the alumni newsletter was updated and increased in size, particularly as more student scholarships and awards were added, and more newsletter space was devoted to articles about the donors and recipients of these scholarships and awards. This increase in the size and sophistication of the newsletter was another indication of the increasing size and reach of the DFM.

In 2009, Puja G. Samudra became the first recipient of the Dale L. Williams, MD, Family Medicine Scholarship. The scholarship is "awarded annually to offset student debt and to recognize an outstanding senior student who has demonstrated a commitment to a career in family medicine and who matches into the U-M Department of Family Medicine residency program. Dr. Williams was on the original committee that presented a proposal to the U-M Board of Regents and the U-M Medical School to develop the Department of Family Medicine. Dr. Williams retired from a private family practice in Muskegon after 30 years and divides his time between Michigan and Florida."

In 2009, David M. Lessens was the first recipient of the Vincent P. and Genevieve L. Burns Family Medicine Scholarship. This scholarship, which was "established by their daughter, Elizabeth (Beth) Burns, MD, a 1976 U-M medical school graduate and family physician, is awarded to a senior medical student based on a combination of outstanding academic achievement, demonstrated financial need, and a commitment to the principles of, and a career in, family medicine."

In 2009, David M. Lessens was also the first recipient of the Chelsea Community Family Medicine Scholarship. This scholarship was "established by a long-time friend and supporter of the Department, Arlene Howe, who played a significant role in establishing the department's inpatient service at Chelsea Community Hospital in 1978. She initiated this scholarship to encourage students to consider family medicine as a specialty. This scholarship is awarded annually to a senior medical student, who has matched into a family medicine residency program, and is based on a combination of outstanding academic and clinical performance and demonstrated financial need." Ms. Howe passed away on August 11, 2017, at the age of ninety-seven. Yet, her legacy lives on in perpetuity through the Chelsea Community Family Medicine Scholarship.

In 2009, Tessa Dake was the initial recipient of the Jill and Thomas R. Berglund, MD, Family Medicine Scholarship. This scholarship is "awarded annually to a senior medical student based on the combination of outstanding academic achievement, demonstrated financial need, and a commitment to the principles of, and a career in, family medicine. Dr. Berglund, who passed away in 2011, was a 1959 UMMS graduate and a family physician in the Kalamazoo area."

In 2010, Lindsey V. Kotagal was the initial recipient of the Alpha Epsilon Iota (AEI) Sorority Family Medicine Scholarship. The scholarship was "established by the designated trustee for the AEI Sorority Fund and family physician, Dr. Marguerite (Peg) Shearer, to support medical students who choose family medicine as their specialty. In 1956, the University of Michigan AEI Sorority was an organization that provided support and encouragement for professional women. As the interest in professional sororities declined and the required maintenance on sorority houses increased, AEI sold their house to the University and placed the money in a trust."

In 2011, Matthew R. Schlough was the initial recipient of the Robert J. Fisher, MD, Family Medicine Scholarship. This scholarship, established in 2010, is "awarded to a senior medical student based on academic achievement, a demonstrated commitment to the principles of, and a career in, family medicine and demonstrated financial need. Dr. Fisher is a 1960 UMMS graduate and, during medical school, he had the honor of serving as the president of his class for three years. He practiced for over 30 years in Ypsi-lanti and sold his practice (now the Ypsilanti Family Medicine Center) to the University upon his retirement."

In the midst of the steady initiation of new scholarships to support student interest in family medicine came the establishment of the George A. Dean, MD, Chair of Family Medicine Fund. A gift of $1.5 million from Dr. Dean marked the establishment of the first endowed professorship in the history of the department. As noted previously, Dr. Dean was intimately involved in the establishment of the department, serving as co-chair of the RPC, which recommended the initial establishment of the department as approved by the Board of Regents in November 1976. Dr. Dean also served on the recruitment committee that identified Terence C. Davies, MD, as the founding chair of the department. Dr. Dean stayed in contact with the department in the intervening years and chose to make this significant financial contribution as part of the University of Michigan's Michigan Difference Campaign. Dr. Dean's gift was supplemented by an additional amount of $500,000 from the Donor Challenge Fund, bringing the total value of the gift to $2 million.

On June 13, 2007, Thomas L. Schwenk, MD, was installed as the first George A. Dean, MD, Chair of Family Medicine in a ceremony in the University Hospital Ford Auditorium. Dean James O. Woolliscroft presided over the ceremony, which included members of the Dean, Davies, and Schwenk families along with department faculty, staff, residents, alumni, and friends. No one could have imagined such an event in the early days of the department, reflecting the remarkable progress made by the department in capitalizing on various opportunities since its establishment.

As noted in chapter 4, the department was first mentioned in National Institutes of Health (NIH) rankings in 1999 when it was ranked third in funding among family medicine departments. The department was first mentioned in the *US News and World Report* (*USNWR*) survey in 2002 as the eighth best family medicine department.

As a frame of reference, in 2007, at the time that Dr. Schwenk was installed as the first George A. Dean, MD, Chair of Family Medicine, the University of Michigan Medical

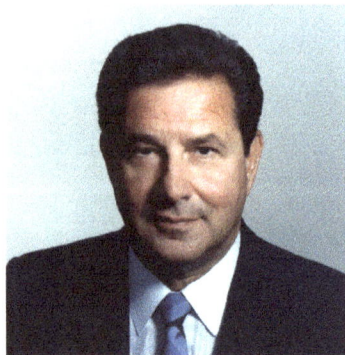

NAME: George A. Dean, MD
ROLE: Major donor who established the endowed chair, The George A. Dean, MD, Chair of Family Medicine
BIO: Co-chair of the RPC and member of the founding chair search committee

Location on March 1, 1978: Southfield, Michigan, seeing patients as a community family physician

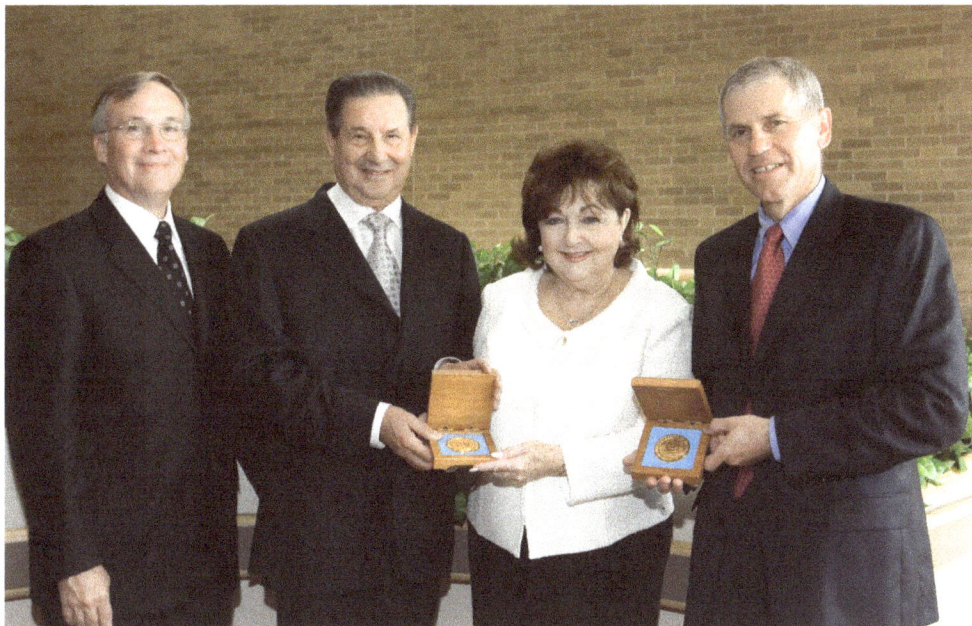

Figure 5.1. June 13, 2007, installation ceremony for Dr. Schwenk as the first George A. Dean, MD, Chair of Family Medicine. *From left to right: Dean Woolliscroft; George A. Dean, MD; Mrs. Vivian Dean; and Thomas L. Schwenk, MD*

School (UMMS) was tied for tenth place in the *USNWR* survey of research-oriented medical schools. In 2007, the DFM was fifth in the rankings of family medicine departments, the highest ranking among all the UMMS departments or specialties for that year and most years since *USNWR* has begun to report those rankings.

In addition to the scholarships and the named professorship, other development efforts helped support initiatives to help preclinical students explore family medicine as a

At some point prior to 2011, Dr. Schwenk invoked the Wolf Credo during one of his State of the Department Addresses (SODA) to exemplify the theme for the coming year. Starting in 2011, the Wolf Credo was added to the summary page of statistics and data that are provided at each SODA.

The Wolf Credo

Respect the elders.
Teach the young.
Cooperate with the pack.
Play when you can.
Hunt when you must.
Rest in between.
Share your affections.
Voice your feelings.
Leave your mark.[1]

career. Donors were able to contribute directly to a fund specifically used to support the Summer Preceptorship Program for UMMS students between the first and second years of medical school. The students were placed with community-based family physicians, all with some sort of alumni connection to the medical school or residency program. The program was designed to provide an early experience in the "real world" of family medicine through caring and competent role models. The first students were placed in the offices of community family physicians in the summer of 2010. Since 2017, this has been referred to as the Kenneth and Judy Betz Summer Preceptorship.

In the second half of this time frame, a new fellowship program was established and some other notable changes were made in leadership positions. More faculty and staff members also received local and national acknowledgment for their efforts. Under the leadership of Dr. Skye, an academic fellowship was established in 2006, combining inpatient and outpatient clinical work with participation in structured development of academic and research skills via programs offered inside and outside the department. Jill N. Fenske, MD, was the first person in this fellowship, which—unlike the existing sports medicine and geriatric fellowships in which the department had long-standing involvement—was not accredited by the Accreditation Council for Graduate Medical Education (ACGME). The lack of ACGME accreditation gave Dr. Skye greater flexibility in some of the options available to him and the fellows in this program. Over the years, a number of the graduates of this program have stayed on as faculty, including Dr. Fenske.

A series of additional fellowships were added in this period. An integrative medicine fellowship was initiated by the department in 2007. Andrew H. Heyman, MD, MHSA, was the first graduate of that fellowship. Two other departments initiated fellowships in conjunction with the DFM over the next two years. The Department of Internal Medicine started the Hospice and Palliative Medicine Fellowship, and J. Brandon Walters, MD, was the first family physician to complete that fellowship in 2008–9. The Department of Obstetrics and Gynecology started the Women's Health Fellowship in 2006, and Ebony C. Parker-Featherstone, MD, was the first family physician to complete that fellowship in 2009–10. As with other fellowships, a number of the graduates stayed on as faculty after completing their fellowship training.

After serving as the initial clerkship director since 1996, Dr. Peggs became the first member of the department to hold a position in the medical school dean's office when he was named assistant dean of student programs in 2007. Joel J. Heidelbaugh, MD, at that time the medical director of the Ypsilanti Health Center, was chosen to be the second clerkship director and continues in that role to this date.

Also in 2007, Dr. Schwenk changed the titles of the existing assistant chairs to associate chairs, with Dr. Peggs's position changing from associate chair to senior associate chair. Dr. Lefever retired in 2007 and was named the department's first emeritus professor, a fitting person for that role as he was the first faculty member hired by Dr. Davies in 1978.

James M. Cooke, MD, was selected as the fifth residency director in 2007 when Dr. Skye assumed the position of assistant chair for educational programs (renamed the associate chair for educational programs as those changes were put into effect).

Earlier in this phase of department history, Quinta Vreede had been chosen as the second department administrator in 2005 to replace Ms. Bomar when she left after fifteen years as the inaugural full-time department administrator. Ms. Vreede served in that role until 2010, when Matthew Bazzani was chosen as her replacement.

For the first thirty-two years of the department's existence, the chair had also served as service chief, with Drs. Davies and Schwenk serving in that role from 1978 to 2010. Given the continuing growth and complexity of the department's position in the health system's inpatient settings, Dr. Schwenk assigned that role to Dr. Chavey in 2010.

Finally, in 2008, Dr. Sheets received the STFM Excellence in Education Award. In 2010, Blythe A. Bieber, the executive administrative assistant to the chair and a staff member since 1979, was acknowledged with the University of Michigan Health System Support Staff of the Year Award. This was the first time a DFM staff member had received such a prestigious honor.

In early 2011, Dr. Schwenk announced that he had accepted the invitation to become dean of the University of Nevada School of Medicine and vice president for Health Sciences at the University of Nevada, Reno. He had joined the department during a time of anxiety regarding the uncertain outcome of an external review and had been its leader through many key moments of the first thirty-three years of its history.

As Dr. Schwenk was completing his time as chair and was preparing to leave for his new position in Reno, he was asked to make a formal presentation to the Dean's Advisory Council (DAC), which included department chairs and administrators, members of the dean's office, and other medical center leaders. Highlights of that March 23, 2011, presentation provide a fitting summary of the twenty-five years from 1986 to 2011 when Dr. Schwenk served as interim chair and chair. The PowerPoint slides from that 2011 DAC presentation provide the content for the following text and tables.[2]

By that point in time, more than 2.5 million patients had been seen by department clinicians, including the delivery of more than 7,500 babies. Cumulative clinical revenue was calculated at $220 million, with $1.2 billion in referral revenue having been generated. At that time, it was estimated that more than 3,600 students had been taught in M3 clerkships and fourth-year (M4) subinternships and electives. There had been 229 residency graduates to date. The department was ranked as the fourth best family medicine department by the *USNWR* methodology, the highest ranked of all medical school departments at UMMS.

Here are the clinical programs identified by Dr. Schwenk as notable in March 2011:

Sports Medicine Consultation Program
Medical Urology

Integrative Medicine Oncology consultations

Family Center Obstetrical and Newborn Care

Japanese Family Health Program

Palliative Care Consultation Program

Adolescent medicine, School-Based Health Care, Corner Health Center

Patient-Centered Medical Home developments

Cielo (originally ClinfoTracker)

Here are the educational programs he similarly identified as notable at that time:

Admissions Committee, FCE (Family-Centered Experience)

M3 Clerkship Ranking

Residency recruitment success

RWJ Clinical Scholars Program

Multidisciplinary fellowships in Palliative Care and Sports Medicine

Educational relative value unit (RVU) program

Family Medicine Educational Scholars Program

Using presentation slides, Dr. Schwenk showed the dramatic growth in the number of faculty members, outpatient visits, work RVUs, inpatient volume, and research expenditures across time frames for which appropriate data were available. Here are the notable research programs Dr. Schwenk identified at that time:

Cancer screening and prevention

Cross-cultural medical care

Women's health

Mental illness in primary care and special populations

Physical activity and chronic disease management in high-risk populations

Physician decision-making and clinical management support

Health information technology

Integrative medicine and alternative therapies

Frailty in the elderly

In nearing the end of his presentation, he listed the following activities as examples of outreach, volunteerism, and community service at the time:

Corner Health Center

School-Based Health Centers

EMU and UM Athletic Medicine

Latino Health Center
Japanese Family Health Center
Migrant farm worker clinic
Hope Clinic
Quito Project
Haiti, Dominican Republic, Jamaica, Ghana

In summarizing the role and visibility of the department outside the institution, he identified the following examples of national leadership and contributions:

ASCCP (American Society for Colposcopy and Cervical Pathology)
JNC VII (The Seventh Report of the Joint National Committee on Prevention, Detection, Evaluation, and Treatment of High Blood Pressure)
NHLBI (National Heart, Lung, and Blood Institute)
NCI (National Cancer Institute)
AAFP (American Academy of Family Physicians)
STFM (Society of Teachers of Family Medicine)
Residency and Department development consultations
Cielo
Institute of Medicine

Another graphic in his presentation summarized the department's national rankings. Rankings for NIH funding within family medicine departments were noted as ranging from third to seventh between 1999 and 2010. Similarly, he listed *USNWR* department rankings between a tie for third to tenth between 2002 and 2011. While he did not include an average ranking on his slide, these rankings equate to an average ranking of 5.3 for NIH funding within family medicine departments and an average ranking of 6.5 among family medicine departments for *USNWR* rankings in those time frames.

In a slide labeled "Not the Small Department It Used to Be," Dr. Schwenk noted that the DFM was now at the median of nineteen UMMS clinical departments in the categories of size of faculty, work RVUs, clinical revenue, research funding, and philanthropy.

In another graphic, he noted collaborations with twenty-two other departments or centers in activities related to patient care, education, and/or research. For eight of the departments or centers, there were activities in patient care, education, and research.

In looking to the future, he spoke about how both the department and the family physician needed to be experts in health care delivery and meet the following criteria:

Population-based
Outcome-driven

Emphasis on chronic disease management and preventive services delivery
Based on the principles of the patient-centered medical home
Dependent on robust and innovative health information technology

The presentation to the DAC provided Dr. Schwenk a large venue of medical school and medical center leaders in which to highlight the progress the department had made since its inception in 1978 and in his twenty-five years as chair. It was an appropriate setting in which to laud department accomplishments and to set the stage for the next phase of the department.

A longstanding tradition among chairs of UMMS departments is to have each chair sign the diploma of each UMMS graduate. A classroom was set up with diplomas on tables so that each chair could come in and easily move from one diploma to another throughout the room and sign in the appropriate spot according to seniority. By the time he signed his last set of diplomas in 2011, Dr. Schwenk was second in seniority. As he was preparing for his move to assume his new position in Reno, he remarked that the diploma he had received when he graduated from medical school in 1975 listed the last chair in terms of seniority to sign his diploma as John J. Vorhees, MD, the professor and chair of the Department of Dermatology. When Dr. Schwenk signed his last set of UMMS diplomas in 2011, the only chair with more seniority was Dr. Vorhees.

As Dr. Schwenk prepared to make his transition from Ann Arbor to Reno, Philip Zazove, MD, was selected by Dean Woolliscroft to serve as interim chair of the DFM. Dr. Zazove began his term as interim chair of the department on June 1, 2011. He had extensive experience in many roles in the department, health system, and medical school since September 1989 on which to base his approach to leadership of a growing academic department with extensive clinical, educational, research, and service missions.

Chapter 5 Timeline: Key Events/Individuals between 2001 and 2011

July 2001	UFP is renamed Family Mother Baby (FMB) Service
2001	Appointment of Eric P. Skye, MD, as vice-chief of medicine service, Chelsea Community Hospital
2002	Fourth residency director: Dr. Skye
2002	Third assistant chair of clinical programs: Jean M. Malouin, MD, MPH
2002	Dr. Schwenk is elected to the Institute of Medicine
2002	First *US News and World Report* (*USNWR*) department ranking: eighth place
2003	First development officer: Amy C. St. Amour
2003	Michael L. Szymanski, MD, is named MAFP Michigan Family Physician of the Year
2003	Dr. Schwenk receives Society of Teachers of Family Medicine (STFM) Recognition Award

2004	Third assistant chair of research: Mack T. Ruffin IV, MD, MPH
2004	Initiation of Department of Family Medicine Senior Scholarship
2004	ClinfoTracker is licensed
2004	Twenty-five-year anniversary event
2005	First scholarship and awards event
2005	Initiation of William Clippert Gorenflo Research Award in Family Medicine
2005	Initiation of Harold Kessler, MD, Scholarship in Family Medicine
2005	Initiation of Kenneth and Judy Betz Family Medicine Scholarship
2005	Initiation of development advisory committee
2005	Second department administrator: Quinta Vreede
2005	Dr. O'Brien is named MAFP Family Medicine Educator of the Year
2006	First assistant chair of information management and quality: Dr. Green
2006	First academic fellow: Jill N. Fenske, MD
2006	East Ann Arbor Health Center site is relocated to Domino's Farms
June 2007	First George A. Dean, MD, Chair of Family Medicine: Dr. Schwenk
2007	Opening of Latino health clinic at Ypsilanti Health Center
2007	First emeritus faculty member: Dr. Lefever
2007	Second clerkship director: Joel J. Heidelbaugh, MD
2007	Fifth residency director: James M. Cooke, MD
2007	Second assistant chair of education: Dr. Skye
2007	Dr. Peggs named assistant dean for student programs
2007	Assistant chairs are redesignated as associate chairs
2007	First senior associate chair: Dr. Peggs
2007	Dr. Skye is named MAFP Family Medicine Educator of the Year
2007	First Integrative Medicine Fellow: Andrew H. Heyman, MD, MHSA
2008	First scholarship and awards luncheon
2008	Thirty-year-anniversary event
2008	First Hospice and Palliative Medicine Fellow: J. Brandon Walters, MD
2008	Dr. Sheets receives STFM Excellence in Education Award
2008	Election of Dr. Skye as chief of staff, Chelsea Community Hospital
2009	Initiation of collaboration with Ghana College of Physicians and Surgeons
2009	Initiation of Dale L. Williams, MD, Family Medicine Scholarship
2009	Initiation of Vincent P. and Genevieve L. Burns Family Medicine Scholarship
2009	Initiation of Chelsea Community Family Medicine Scholarship

2009	Initiation of Jill and Thomas R. Berglund, MD, Family Medicine Scholarship
2009	First Women's Health Fellow: Ebony C. Parker-Featherstone, MD
2010	Initiation of Alpha Epsilon Iota (AEI) Sorority Family Medicine Scholarship
2010	Third department administrator: Matthew Bazzani
2010	Third service chief: William E. Chavey II, MD
2010	Blythe A. Bieber is selected as recipient of University of Michigan's Health System Support Staff of the Year Award
2010	Initiation of Summer Preceptorship Program
2011	Initiation of Robert J. Fisher, MD, Family Medicine Scholarship

6

2011 to 2017
Maintaining Our Position While Continuing to Move Forward

D r. Zazove has long brought a different set of credentials and experience to the Department of Family Medicine (DFP) leadership, although his position there was not clear from the outset. Like Dr. Davies, he was married to another family physician, but in this instance, he was the "trailing" spouse when Dr. Schwenk recruited his wife, Dr. Reed, to come bolster the faculty's research faculty ranks in 1989. Dr. Schwenk recalled in an interview conducted in 2015 that it was not clear at the time of Dr. Reed's recruitment what Dr. Zazove would do once he got to Ann Arbor. After exploring some other options outside the department and family medicine, Dr. Zazove joined the faculty in September 1989 as a clinical assistant professor involved in a variety of roles across all department missions. In addition to being named the first assistant chair of clinical programs in 1995, he was also the first faculty member appointed to a major clinical leadership position outside the department when he was named west region medical director within ambulatory care services of the health system in 1997. He continued to serve in other leadership roles within ambulatory care services and M-CARE, along with serving on the medical school executive committee from 2007 to 2010. He also found time between 1992 and 1994 to commute to Evanston to get a master's degree in management from his undergraduate alma mater, Northwestern University.

In June 2011, he began his term as interim chair. After a national search that brought three external candidates to Ann Arbor for interviews and presentations, Dr. Zazove was selected to be the third chair in the history of the department and was installed as the

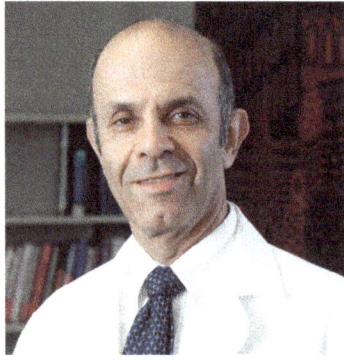

NAME: Philip Zazove, MD
ROLE: Third chair and second George A. Dean, MD, Chair
BIO: Previously at University of Utah, faculty member in DFM since 1989

Location on March 1, 1978: St. Louis, Missouri, on a fourth-year ophthalmology clerkship awaiting couples match results

second George A. Dean, MD, Chair of Family Medicine, with that appointment beginning on December 1, 2012.

In addition to the successful establishment of the George A. Dean, MD, Chair of Family Medicine position in 2007, other development efforts in that same time period resulted in the establishment of an endowed research professor position. In November 2011, Mack T. Ruffin IV, MD, MPH, was installed as the first Dr. Max and Buena Lichter Research Professor of Family Medicine, a position that was "established in 2007 through a generous gift from Dr. Allen and Evie Lichter and Dr. Paul and Carolyn Lichter. This professorship honors the memory of their father, Dr. Max Lichter, a family physician who practiced in Melvindale, a Detroit suburb, for five decades and their mother, Buena Lichter, and is intended to encourage and support research in family medicine." Dr. Allen Lichter served as professor and chair of the Department of Radiation Oncology and dean of the University of Michigan Medical School (UMMS), and his brother, Dr. Paul Lichter, served as professor and chair of the Department of Ophthalmology during much of Dr. Schwenk's term as chair.

In 2012, Lee A. Green, MD, MPH, was named chair of the University of Alberta Department of Family Medicine. Dr. Green became the first residency graduate to become a department chair and also became the third emeritus faculty member.

More student scholarships also made their debuts during this phase. In 2012, Angeline Ti was the first recipient of the Paddy and Donald N. Fitch, MD, Family Medicine Scholarship. (A complete list of recipients of this scholarship and others mentioned in the chapter is included in appendix D.) This scholarship was "established in 2011 and is awarded to a senior medical student based on academic achievement, a demonstrated commitment to the principles of, and a career in, family medicine and demonstrated financial need. Dr. Fitch, a family physician, graduated from U-M Medical School in 1959 and practiced in Escanaba, Michigan. He passed away in August of 2011."

In 2015, Yorgos E. Strangas was the initial recipient of the Michael Papo, MD, Family Medicine Scholarship, which is "awarded annually to a senior medical student based on the combination of outstanding academic achievement, demonstrated financial need, and

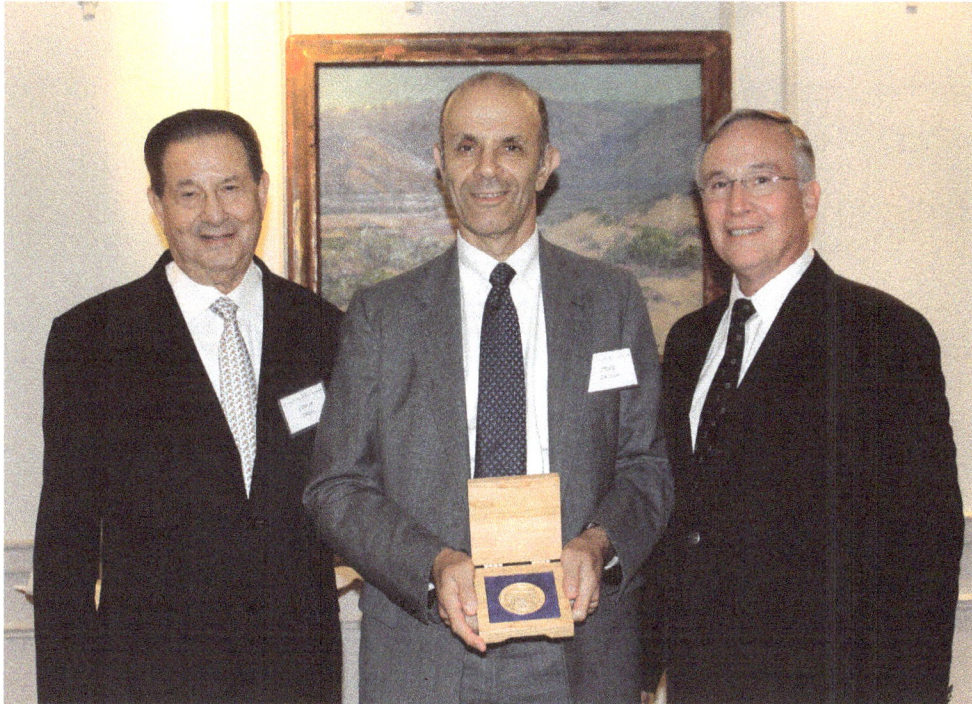

Figure 6.1. 2012 installation of Dr. Zazove as the second George A. Dean, MD, Chair of Family Medicine. *From left to right: Dr. Dean, Dr. Zazove, and Dean Woolliscroft*

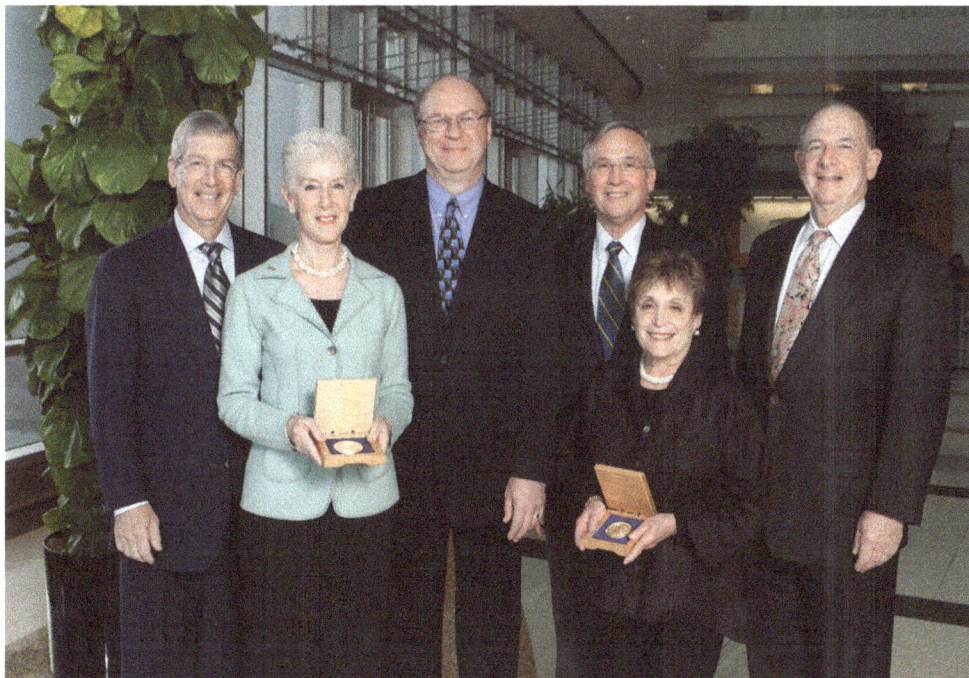

Figure 6.2. 2011 installation ceremony for Dr. Ruffin as the first Lichter Research Professor. *From left to right: Allen S. Lichter, MD; Mrs. Evie S. Lichter; Mack T. Ruffin IV, MD, MPH; Dean Woolliscroft; Mrs. Carolyn R. Lichter; and Dr. Paul R. Lichter*

a commitment to the principles of, and a career in, family medicine. Dr. Papo passed away in November of 2012." Dr. Papo played a key role in the efforts of local and state-wide family physicians to establish the Department of Family Practice at the University of Michigan. Dr. Papo and his classmate from the UMMS class of 1957, James Botsford, MD, started a practice in downtown Chelsea in 1958 after they completed rotating internships. Later Drs. Papo and Botsford relocated to a new building, the Chelsea Medical Clinic, farther south down Main Street in 1966. In 1978, that building was rented and later purchased by the University and became the first clinical site for the new department when it formally started on March 1, 1978. Dr. Papo also led the effort to establish Chelsea Community Hospital, which continues to be a critical partner in the department's educational and clinical missions to this date.

In 2016, Jonathan Waldmann was the first recipient of the Gazella-Brandle Memorial Family Medicine Scholarship, which was "established by Gary R. Gazella, MD, in honor and memory of Dr. Gazella's sister, Kathy Lynn Gazella; Dr. Gazella's father, Richard LaVern Gazella; and Dr. Gazella's mother-in-law, Doris Arlen Hanson Brandle. It is awarded annually to a senior medical student based on the combination of outstanding academic achievement, demonstrated financial need, and a commitment to the principles of, and a career in, family medicine."

In all, at the most recent scholarship and award event in May 2017, more than $80,000 was given to residents and medical students, a significant increase from the $20,000 given to students in 2004 when the first scholarships were awarded.

In addition to the efforts to establish additional student scholarships, the first lectureships were also established in this era. The Terence C. Davies, MD, Endowed Lectureship in Medical Education was established in 2014, and the first two visiting lecturers that were brought back to campus were familiar figures in the department. Dr. Schwenk returned from Nevada in 2014 to give the initial presentation, and in 2015, Dr. Green returned from Canada to give the second presentation in this series. (A list of details on these lectures and others mentioned in this chapter is provided in appendix F.) This endowment was created to support "an annual lectureship in family medicine that will feature a prominent speaker and family medicine educator, who embodies the same values and passion that Terry exemplified as Chair of the Department."

A second lectureship was initiated in July 2015. The Drs. Earl and Louise Zazove Lectureship in Family Medicine was established in honor of Dr. Zazove's parents. There have been three Zazove Lectures to date, all focusing in some fashion on issues related to the study of aging, as its purpose statement requires: "The Drs. Earl and Louise Zazove Lectureship in Family Medicine will support an annual lectureship in family medicine and an education program focused on aging that will feature a prominent speaker and family medicine educator."

Changes in leadership positions and the bestowal of faculty accolades continued during this time period. In 2012, Grant M. Greenberg, MD, MSHA, MA, was appointed to replace Dr. Green as associate chair for information management and quality. Also in 2012, Dr. Cooke stepped down as residency director and was named executive director of the University of Michigan Health System (UMHS) Clinical Simulation Center. This represented the first appointment of this kind in department history. After a period of time with Tarannum A. Master-Hunter, MD, serving as interim residency director, Margaret L. Dobson, MD, was named as the sixth residency director in 2013. That same year, David C. Serlin, MD, was appointed to succeed Dr. Malouin as associate chair for clinical programs.

Outside the department and the institution, Randall T. Forsch, MD, MPH, was named chief medical officer of Chelsea Community Hospital. This was the most significant appointment of a faculty member within the administrative structure of the department's longtime partnership with Chelsea Community Hospital in providing care in the greater Chelsea community.

Several faculty members received accolades during the early years of Dr. Zazove's leadership. Stefani A. Hudson, MD, was the second faculty member to receive the MAFP Michigan Family Physician Award in 2012. Dr. Peggs was inducted into the inaugural class of the UMMS League of Clinical Excellence in 2012. Also in 2012, Dr. Reed received the Physician Mentorship Recognition Award from the American Medical Association Women Physicians Congress. In 2013, Sara L. Warber, MD, was awarded a Fulbright Scholarship, the first department member to have received this prestigious recognition while a member of the faculty.

Over this period, progress and challenges continued across department missions. The implementation of MiChart as a new outpatient electronic medical record system in August 2012 served as one example, causing a great deal of stress on faculty, residents, fellows, and staff in the process of caring for patients and teaching students and residents in the outpatient setting. The challenge of procuring and maintaining sufficient space to accommodate the personnel needed to pursue department missions has remained another consistent issue through the history of the DFM. From the original administrative space adjacent to the animal labs to the space in the Clinical Faculty Office Building to 1018 Fuller to the space in Women's Hospital, the location of the department has been the subject of negotiations regarding space in the agenda of each of the three chairs. With the appointment of Dr. Zazove as the third chair in 2012, the pursuit of more suitable space moved from a "to-do" list item to action. And through a remarkable series of decisions made at upper levels in the medical center administration, space became available on the seventh floor of Medical Science I, the same space where the dean's office was housed during the early years of the department. Many critical letters and memos used as contemporaneous documents in writing this history originated from this same space in the 1970s and 1980s.

Over Memorial Day weekend of 2013, the faculty and staff members who had been based in Women's Hospital since 1999 were relocated to the seventh-floor suite along with other faculty and staff who had remained in the 1018 Fuller building. While there was not enough room for the research faculty and staff and some general administrative staff to make the move to the suite, the new location did open room for some new faculty and staff associated with research mission efforts to move into 1018 Fuller. The symbolism of the move to the seventh (and top) floor of Medical Science Building I was apparent through the medical center. As Dr. Lefever emailed at the time of the move, the department had gone from "the doghouse to the penthouse" in the thirty-five years since its inception.

A celebration of the first thirty-five years of the department was held in April 2014. Dr. Davies—who had also returned for the events in 1998, 2004, and 2008—and Dr. Schwenk attended, and both made formal comments along with Dr. Zazove and others. Many former faculty, residency program and medical school graduates, and other friends of the department assembled for the celebration, which included a gathering of resident graduates in an informal setting on Friday evening followed by a more formal event on Saturday evening. The size and scope of these events and the number of participants would have been inconceivable in 1978, much less in 1982 or 1988 when the initial celebrations of the department were held.

The department's focus on education was acknowledged in 2013 when four faculty members, Drs. Cooke, Peggs, Sheets, and Skye, were all inducted into the inaugural class of the UMMS League of Educational Excellence. In 2016, four more department faculty

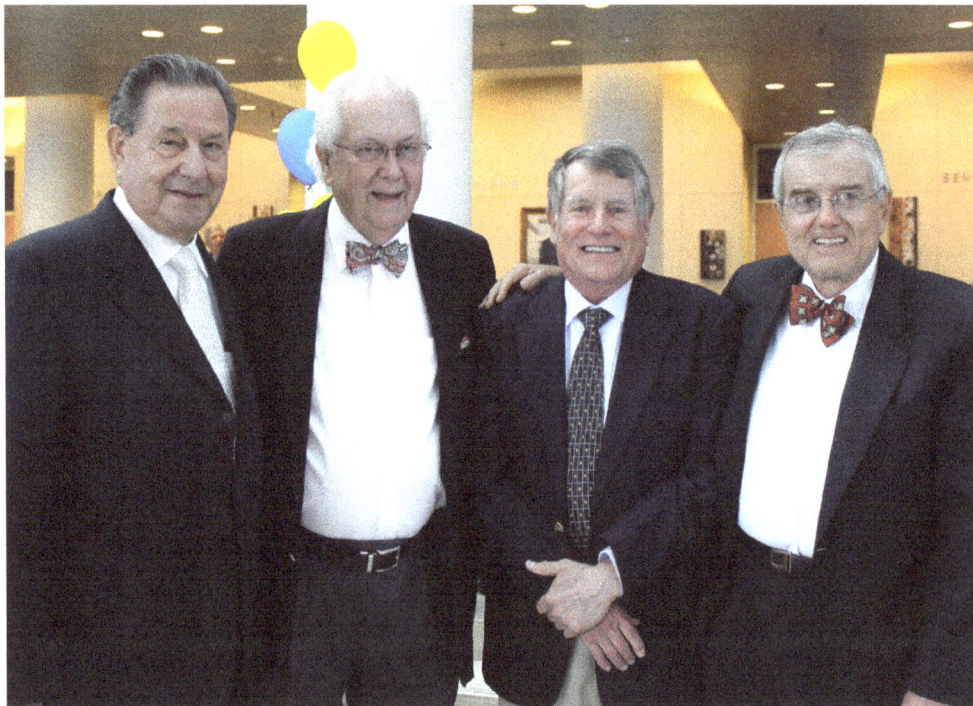

Figure 6.3. Dr. Davies and original members of the 1975–76 Residency Planning Committee in April 2014. *From left to right: Dr. Dean; Dr. Davies; Gary R. Gazella, MD; and Dale L. Williams, MD*

were inducted into the league: Kristina M. Gallagher, MD; Dr. Heidelbaugh; Margaret A. Riley, MD; and Pamela G. Rockwell, DO.

In 2014, Dr. Sheets received the UMMS Lifetime Achievement Award in Medical Education, and in 2015, Dr. Skye was named one of four learning community directors within the structure of the new UMMS curriculum. In the same year, within the research mission, Dr. Ruffin was inducted into the UMMS League of Research Excellence, and Ananda Sen, PhD, received a Collegiate Research Professorship Award.

Just as Dr. Green had left to become chair of a department elsewhere, Dr. Ruffin left in 2016 to become chair of the Department of Family and Community Medicine at the Penn State University Hershey Medical Center. Caroline R. Richardson, MD, replaced him as associate chair for research programs and was also named the second Dr. Max and Buena Lichter Research Professor of Family Medicine.

Dr. Greenberg also left in 2016 when he was named chair of the Department of Family Medicine at the Lehigh Valley Health Network in Allentown, Pennsylvania. He was replaced on an interim basis as associate chair for information management and quality by Heather Holmstrom, MD, before she left in 2017 for a position at the University of Colorado in Denver. The position was renamed as the associate chair for population management, assumed by Kathryn M. Harmes, MD, in 2017.

In 2017, the residency program began to initiate a "Clinic First" approach to residency education that would prioritize ambulatory care and continuity of care practice over

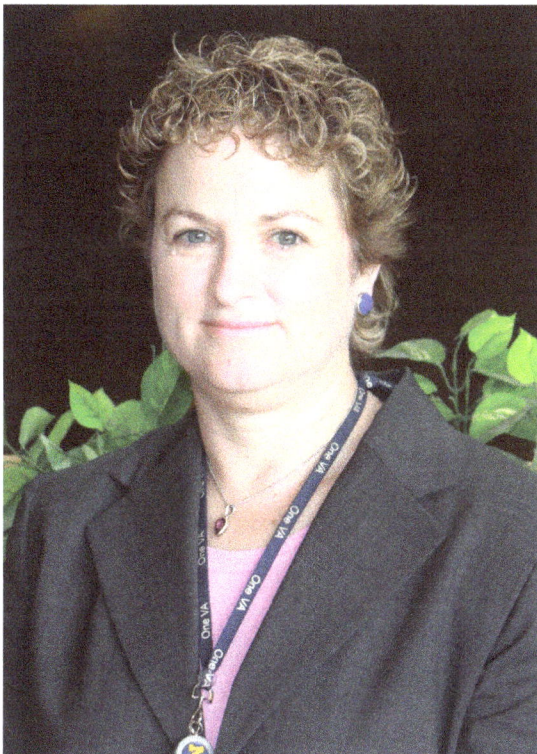

Figure 6.4. Caroline R. Richardson, MD

Endowed Chairs and Professors as of October 1, 2017
George A. Dean, MD, Chair of Family Medicine
Thomas L. Schwenk, MD, 2007 to 2011
Philip Zazove, MD, 2012 to Present

Dr. Max and Buena Lichter Research Professor of Family Medicine
Mack T. Ruffin IV, MD, MPH, 2011 to 2016
Caroline R. Richardson, MD, 2016 to present

inpatient care. The program was also authorized to recruit thirteen residents per class beginning with the incoming class of June 2018, a significant increase from the class of four who started in July 1979.

Three faculty members were honored at the 2017 Society of Teachers of Family Medicine's (STFM) annual spring conference in San Diego. Anne L. Kittendorf, MD, received the STFM Advocate Award, and Margaret A. Riley, MD, received the STFM Innovative Program Award. Emeritus faculty member Mack T. Ruffin IV, MD, MPH, was the recipient of the Curtis G. Hames Research Award.

In the summer of 2017, word came that it was time for the department to move its administrative offices yet again. Planning began for moving the department administrative offices from the seventh-floor suite in Medical Science Building I to the fourth floor of the 300 North Ingalls Building, which had been the site of St. Joseph Mercy Hospital until 1977.

As noted near the end of chapter 5, Dr. Schwenk gave a talk to the Dean's Advisory Council in March 2011 in which he highlighted a number of the accomplishments of the department from 1978 to 2011. Those accomplishments are summarized in the text and in tables 5.1 to 5.5.

In July 2017, Dr. Zazove reviewed the PowerPoint slides from that presentation and provided a written document in which he noted additional accomplishments that had occurred or been enhanced in the six years since Dr. Schwenk's presentation.[1]

Here are the additional clinical programs identified by Dr. Zazove (in addition to those listed in chapter 5) as notable in July 2017:

MiPCT (Michigan Primary Care Transformation Project)
Scribes
Pre-visits
Quality and Guidelines Leadership
C-Sections Conducted by Family Physicians

Here are the educational programs he similarly identified as notable at that time:

Residency expansion

Medical student program leadership in new curriculum (MHome, Branches)

Multiple new fellowships

Clinical Simulation Center Leadership

Ongoing Highly Rated Continuing Medical Education Programs

Here are additional notable research programs identified by Dr. Zazove in July 2017:

Disabilities

Mixed Methods

Health Literacy

Substance Abuse

In addition to the extensive examples that Dr. Schwenk listed as evidence of outreach, volunteerism, and community service in 2011, many of which continue to this date, Dr. Zazove added the community of Flint and the Deaf population to the long list. He also added the Association of Departments of Family Medicine and multiple specialty organizations such as the International Society for the Study of Vulvovaginal Disease, the Society of Decision-Making, and the Association of Medical Professionals with Hearing Losses to the list of national leadership and contributions in chapter 5. In regard to research, Dr. Zazove identified new research collaborations in three of the twenty-two departments or centers identified by Dr. Schwenk six years earlier.

In looking to the future, Dr. Zazove added three new items in bold print to Dr. Schwenk's 2011 list of health care delivery criteria: an emphasis on quality and maximized value, the address of population health in addition to individuals, and evidence-based work.

In the previous chapter, information was provided regarding averages for NIH and *USNWR* department rankings up through 2011. These average rankings are now updated with data available as of September 2017. Rankings for NIH funding within family medicine departments ranged from third to twelfth between 1999 and 2017. *USNWR* department rankings ranged from a tie for third to tenth between 2002 and 2017. These rankings equated to an average ranking of 5.4 for NIH funding and an average ranking of 5.8 for *USNWR* rankings.

On September 13, 2017, the most recent SODA presentation was given by Dr. Zazove. The entire 2017 SODA "report card" is included in appendix H. One notable highlight is the size of the department in terms of human resources statistics: 99 faculty, 290 staff, 33 residents, and 12 fellows.

At this point in time, considering all the clinical activity between 1978 and September 2017, more than 3.2 million patient visits had been documented by department clinicians, including the delivery of more than 10,900 babies. At this time, it was estimated that more than 5,300 students had been taught in family medicine clinical clerkships, subinternships, and electives. There had been 289 residency graduates. The department was tied for the fourth best family medicine department by the *USNWR* methodology, the highest ranked of all medical school departments at the UMMS. The estimated NIH ranking among family medicine departments across the nation was sixth. The total research grant funding for 2016–17, including direct and indirect costs, was over $3.5 million. The total research grant funding from 1978 to 2017 was over $60 million.

As the period of time covered by this book draws near present day, new opportunities and uncertainties regarding the short-term and long-term priorities of the department across missions need to be recognized and addressed. In 2016, Dr. Zazove commissioned Dr. Lefever to work with department leadership to fashion a strategic plan to guide the department moving forward. As of early October 2017, the faculty leaders and groups had completed the plan and now are fully engaged in the important implementation process.

In an email communication, Dr. Lefever summarized the strategic plan in this fashion:

With the intent to create, not predict, our future, the department leadership has confirmed ten (10) goals across all department missions:

Education—(1) students and residents will experience the essential elements of providing comprehensive family medicine, while training in our practices, and faculty will identify and educate learners on these shared, core components; (2) a well-defined cohort of residency-focused faculty will be identified and serve as the core faculty for our residency training program; and, (3) strategies for impacting the overarching medical education experience/curriculum for all medical students will be developed to assure family medicine input and influence.

Research—(1) position the Department as one of the top, three research programs in family medicine at the national level; and, (2) move the Mixed Methods Research Group and the Disability Research Group toward official recognition as research centers with institutional support and national recognition.

Medical Care—(1) position the Department as a national leader in exemplifying family medicine care delivery, developing a model that enhances the patient's experience and maximizes physician satisfaction; and, (2) pursue collaborative opportunities and projects with other primary care departments/divisions to develop an advocacy group for primary care influence.

Advocacy—(1) develop sustainable, department processes that promote diversity, equity and inclusion and support our commitment to recruit and retain diverse talent such that faculty members, residents and staff "mirror" the diversity of the communities we serve; and, (2) increase the "joy of practice" and decrease "burnout" rate to be at or below the national rate for non-physician professionals.

Faculty Development—intentionally invest in faculty development to ensure the department's core interests and commitments are continuously supported through the development of a "pipeline" of leaders and area experts.[2]

The department and its leaders have proven to be resilient and perseverant throughout its history, and using the most recent strategic plan to guide future development, they will continue the tradition and processes followed since 1978.

Chapter 6 Timeline: Key Events/Individuals between 2011 and 2017

2011	Dr. Schwenk accepts position at the University of Nevada
2011	Dr. Zazove is named interim chair
2011	First Dr. Max and Buena Lichter Research Professor of Family Medicine: Dr. Ruffin
2012	Second associate chair for information management and quality: Grant M. Greenberg, MD, MSHA, MA
2012	Stefani A. Hudson, MD, is named MAFP Michigan Family Physician of the Year
2012	Dr. Cooke is named executive director of University of Michigan Health System (UMHS) Clinical Simulation Center
2012	Dr. Peggs is inducted into inaugural class of UMMS League of Clinical Excellence
2012	Dr. Reed receives Physician Mentorship Recognition Award from the American Medical Association Women Physicians Congress
2012	Initiation of Paddy and Donald N. Fitch, MD, Family Medicine Scholarship
August 2012	Implementation of MiChart, outpatient electronic medical record
2012	Dr. Zazove is appointed third department chair and second George A. Dean, MD, chair
May 2013	Move from Women's to the Medical Science I seventh-floor suite
2013	Sixth residency director: Margaret L. Dobson, MD
2013	Fourth associate chair of clinical programs: David C. Serlin, MD
2013	Sara L. Warber, MD, is awarded Fulbright Scholarship
2013	Drs. Cooke, Peggs, Sheets, and Skye are inducted into inaugural class of UMMS League of Educational Excellence
2013	Dr. Peggs is awarded the MAFP Archie Award of Excellence

2013	Kathrine J. Gold, MD, MSW, MS, is selected as the James C. Puffer, MD/American Board of Family Medicine fellow at the National Academy of Medicine
2013	Randall T. Forsch, MD, MPH, is named chief medical officer of Chelsea Community Hospital
April 2014	Thirty-five-year anniversary event
2014	Initiation of Terence C. Davies, MD, Endowed Lectureship in Medical Education
2014	Dr. Sheets receives UMMS Lifetime Achievement Award in Medical Education
2014	Dr. Skye is named director of Path of Excellence Program within new UMMS curriculum
2014	Appointment of Stephen M. Wampler, MD, as vice-chief of Medicine Service, Chelsea Community Hospital
2015	Dr. Skye is named one of four MHome learning community directors within new UMMS curriculum
2015	Caroline R. Richardson, MD, joins leadership team of Institute for Healthcare Policy and Innovation
2015	Dr. Ruffin is inducted into UMMS League of Research Excellence
2015	Ananda Sen, PhD, receives Collegiate Research Professorship Award
2015	Dr. Kiningham is awarded American Medical Society of Sports Medicine Founders' Award
2015	Dr. Zazove is featured on CNN's *The Human Factor*
2015	Initiation of Michael Papo, MD, Family Medicine Scholarship
July 2015	Initiation of Drs. Earl and Louise Zazove Lectureship in Family Medicine
2016	Initiation of Gazella-Brandle Memorial Family Medicine Scholarship
2016	Approval of Brighton Health Center
2016	Fourth associate chair for research programs: Dr. Richardson
2016	Second Dr. Max and Buena Lichter Research Professor of Family Medicine: Dr. Richardson
2016	Third associate chair of information management and quality (interim): Heather L. Holmstrom, MD
2016	Michael D. Fetters, MD, MPH, MA, serves as Fulbright Distinguished Chair of Social Sciences at Peking University Health Sciences Center
2016	Initiation of the Mixed Methods Research and Scholarship Program by Dr. Fetters and John W. Creswell, PhD
2017	Summer preceptorship formally is named the Kenneth and Judy Betz Summer Preceptorship

2017	First associate chair for population medicine (formerly Information Management and Quality): Kathryn M. Harmes, MD
2017	Approved expansion of residency class size to thirteen
2017	Announcement of move to 300 North Ingalls building
April 2018	Fortieth-year anniversary event

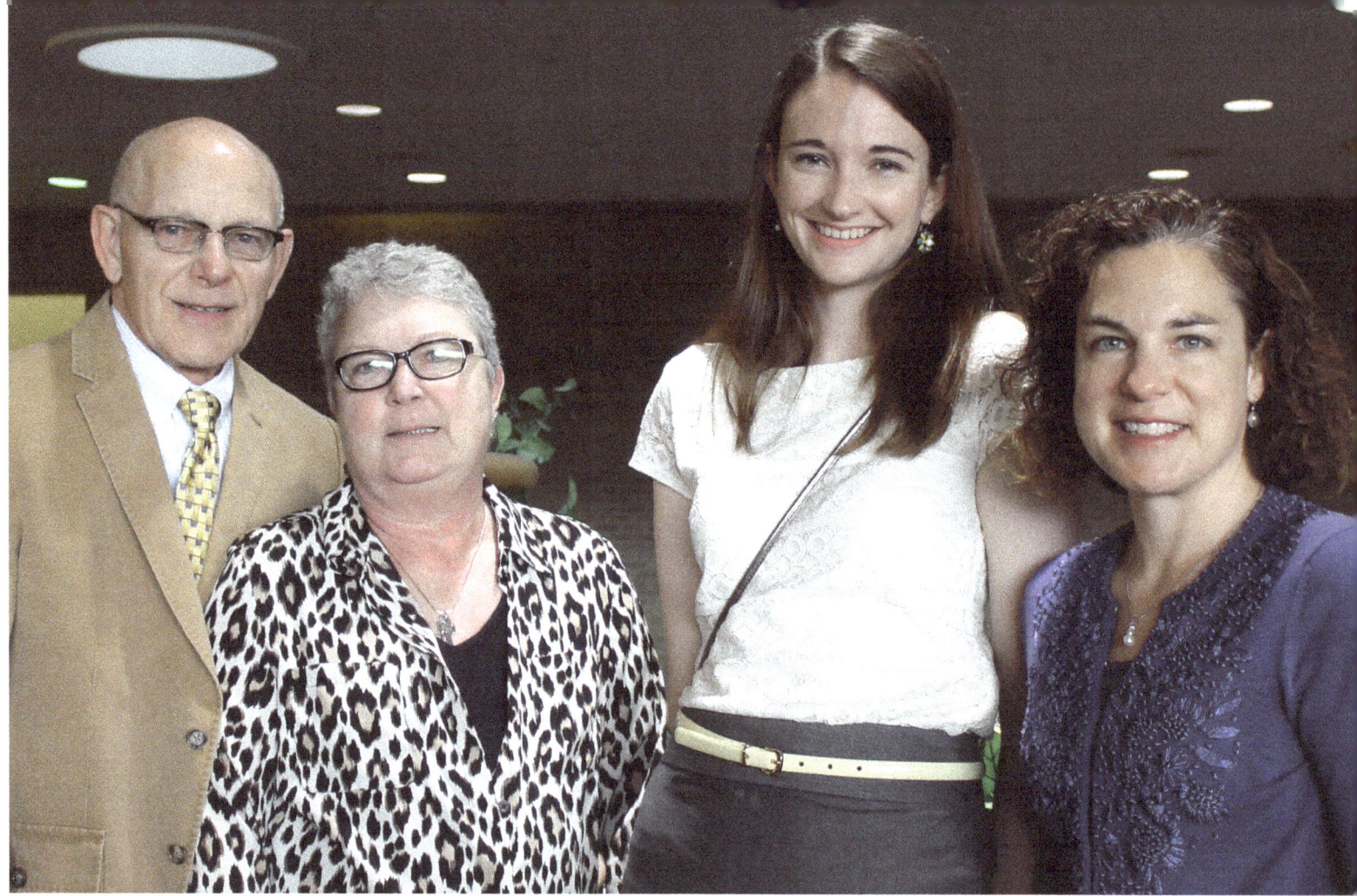
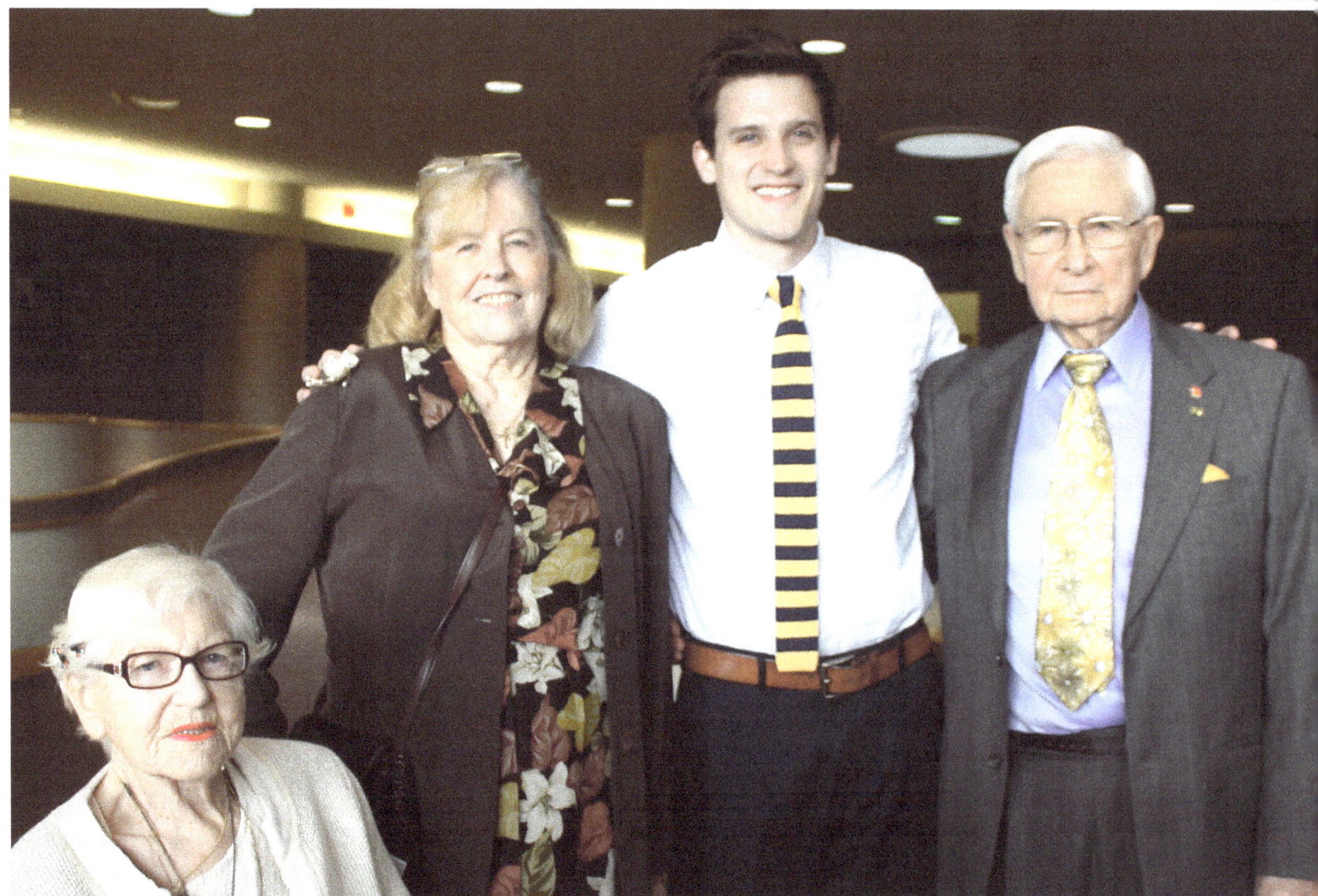

7

2017 and Beyond
Summary and Lessons
Learned along the Way

As with many things, retrospection offers one the opportunity to examine the past, providing greater clarity to the present. When looking over the past forty years of family medicine at the University of Michigan, it is easy to see how certain things that were true in 1978 have continued to be so in 1988, 1998, 2008, and 2017 and likely will continue for many decades to come. The planning priorities from the July 1978 document mentioned in chapter 2 are still applicable in October 2017. In a similar fashion, some of the comments made by Dr. Davies and others early in the history of the department have turned out to be accurate in forecasting the potential for doing work this important in a place as prestigious as the University of Michigan.

As a reminder, here are the July 1978 planning priorities:

A. Stabilize and develop patient-care at the Family Practice Center for further equipping, renovating and extending of present facilities. Resolve those identified problems which are present within the Family Practice Center. Work on community relations and patient education concerning Family Practice.
B. Complete an Affiliation Agreement with the Chelsea Community Hospital.
C. Complete a curriculum proposal for the Family Practice Residency Program in collaboration with all major departments in the Medical College.
D. Seek further funding (Kellogg Foundation, HEW, etc.) for special program development.
E. Recruit needed faculty.

F. Identify and develop teaching input into the undergraduate curriculum (including individual student needs, electives and "core" curricula).

G. Further develop research goals and protocols and prioritize research ambitions.

H. Continue and develop collaborative efforts for Continuing Medical Education for Family Physicians.

I. Plan a sequence of faculty development exercises.[1]

While some of these specific items are not as important or relevant as others in 2017, most of the activities and mission areas included on the list are still highly important and relevant now and will continue to be so moving forward.

In looking back across the past thirty-nine years plus of accomplishments and contributors, many key moments and themes emerged. Many of the things that intrigued Dr. Davies about the possibilities of potential greatness associated with tackling the task of starting an academic family medicine department in a highly subspecialized environment have proven to be similar for Drs. Schwenk and Zazove in subsequent eras. Likewise, some of the challenges encountered by Dr. Davies did not suddenly disappear for the next two chairs and are not likely to disappear for future chairs.

The value of being perseverant and the ability to respond to opportunities as they arise have been common themes across the entire life span of the department. The importance of supportive leadership and peers is equally relevant. In more recent years, the key role of donors has emerged as a large component of the success of the department that was not conceivable in the earliest days, but the department's focus on trust, respect, competence, and achievement laid the foundation for this key role from day one. People in higher levels of authority at the University of Michigan might not always fully understand what family physicians can do in their roles as academic clinicians, educators, and researchers, but it is hard to disregard the level of accomplishment illustrated by department rankings as determined by the NIH, *USNWR*, and student ratings of required clerkships.

The University of Michigan Medical School (UMMS) has proven to be both a challenging and a fertile environment for the Department of Family Medicine. Before there was a department, there were large numbers of UMMS graduates choosing to go into family practice residency programs around the state and nation. The fact that many of them were leaving the state for residency training and practice was part of the impetus for the state legislature and the Michigan Academy of Family Physicians (MAFP) to lobby for academic departments and residency programs to be established at the three allopathic medical schools at the University of Michigan, Michigan State University (MSU), and Wayne State University in the 1970s. Considering the leadership roles played by UMMS graduates after the department was established in 1978, it is clear why "leaders" is a key word in the school fight song.

Before there was a chance to do postgraduate work in family medicine at the University of Michigan, many future department chairs, residency directors, and leaders of health care systems and family medicine graduated from UMMS and went elsewhere to do rotating internships, general practice residency, or family practice residency training. Among the many future leaders who graduated from medical school in Ann Arbor, one key graduate returned to town and became chair for twenty-five years, then became dean of a medical school in another state. Two of the chairs of the Department of Family Medicine at the MSU College of Human Medicine have been UMMS grads, as was a longtime chair at the Medical College of Ohio (now University of Toledo). A recent chair at the University of Virginia was a classmate of Dr. Schwenk in medical school. Someone a year behind Dr. Schwenk served as chair at several medical schools and as an associate dean and now serves as the president of a college in Detroit. There is most definitely something in the air or water in Ann Arbor that attracts people to come here as students, residents, fellows, and faculty. Whether they stay or move on, many of them do great things as leaders in many kinds of settings.

The careers of the first four graduates of the residency program foreshadow much of what was to come in terms of the outcomes of the graduates who would follow in their footsteps. Scott H. Frank, MD, MS, left the state in July 1982 and has not returned. He went to Case Western Reserve University in Cleveland to complete a Robert Wood Johnson Fellowship and complete his MS degree in family medicine. He has stayed at Case Western ever since in a variety of faculty roles, serving for eighteen years as the founding director of their MPH degree program. Recently, he shifted roles to become director of public health initiatives in the Department of Population and Quantitative Health Sciences. He also received fellowship training in addiction medicine along the way and served as a residency director and director of predoctoral education among his other faculty leadership roles.

Patrick J. Kearney, MD, also left the state in 1982 and has not returned, spending four years in the Indian Health Service in Shiprock, New Mexico, prior to taking a position in Durango, Colorado, where he continues to practice full-spectrum family medicine in the community setting. He is a past president of the medical staff at Mercy Regional Medical Center in Durango, and since 2011, he has been a member of the medical staff of Open Sky Wilderness Therapy.

John M. O'Brien, MD, never left the county, much less the state. He stayed on as faculty in the department and has been practicing in Chelsea since his first day as an intern in July 1979. He served as residency director for sixteen years and has worked in a range of other teaching and administrative capacities, including delivering hundreds of babies and caring for adolescent patients in middle schools and other settings in eastern Washtenaw County, along with his outpatient practice in Chelsea.

Fred J. Van Alstine, MD, MBA, also remained in the state for all of his clinical practice, leaving it temporarily to get additional specialized training beyond his family medicine residency experience. He started in community practice in Durand, Michigan, in 1982 and later moved to nearby Owosso. Dr. Van Alstine got his pilot's license, enabling

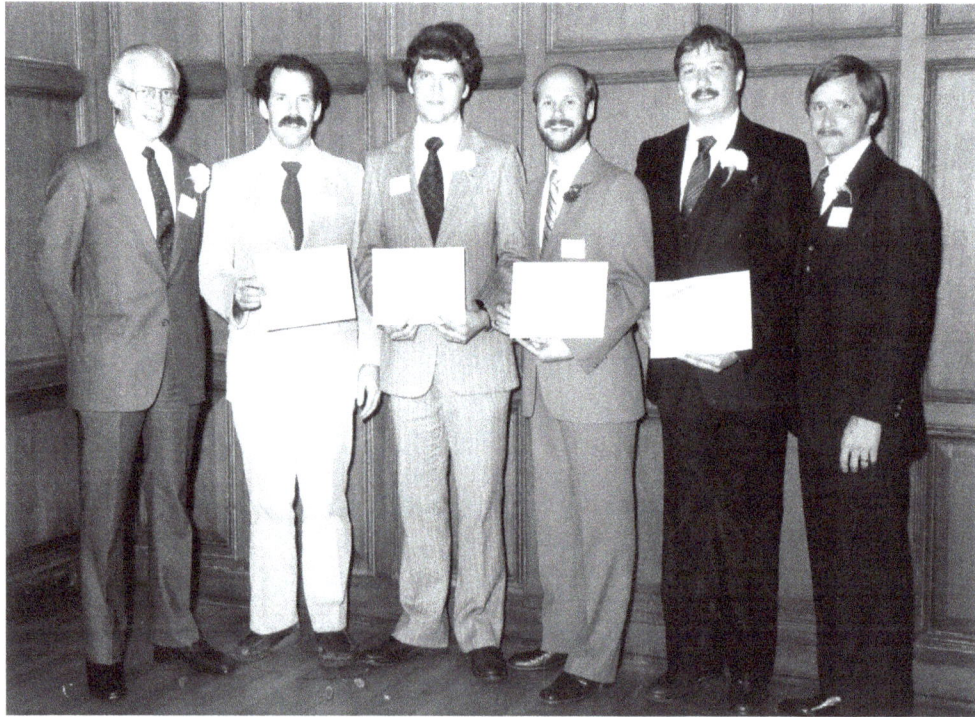

Figure 7.1. Graduation ceremony for the first class of residents in 1982. *From left to right: Dr. Davies, Dr. Frank, Dr. O'Brien, Dr. Kearney, Dr. Van Alstine, and Dr. Peggs*

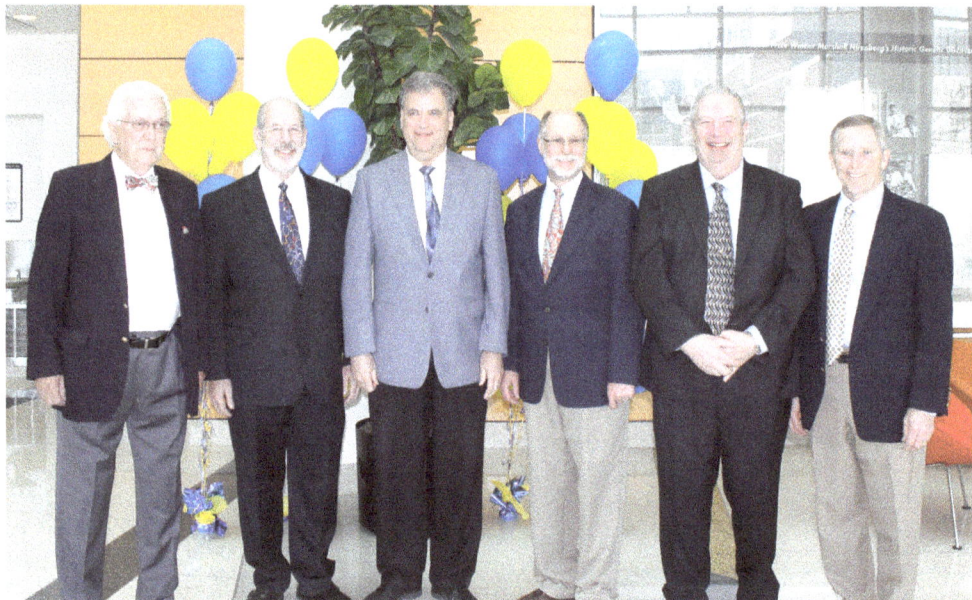

Figure 7.2. Reunion of the first class of residents in 2014. *From left to right: Dr. Davies, Dr. Frank, Dr. O'Brien, Dr. Kearney, Dr. Van Alstine, and Dr. Peggs*

him to pursue educational programs out of state. He completed an MBA in Chicago and a hospice and palliative care fellowship in Atlanta. He also served as president of the Michigan Academy of Family Physicians in 2013–14. In July 2017, he moved to Gaylord, Michigan, and began to use his palliative care training for the Munson Healthcare System in Traverse City.

Across the diverse career paths of the four original graduates, one can see how the department and residency program have contributed to the care of patients in settings that span the scope of family medicine. Little did anyone know in June 1982 who or what was to become of this experiment in family medicine at the University of Michigan, but these four pioneers certainly used their education and training as medical students and family practice residents to go on paths that reflect the options that can be pursued by individuals who choose to enter family medicine at the University of Michigan.

In addition to the diverse career paths taken by the 289 residency graduates between 1982 and 2017, the diversity of the composition of the residents has changed dramatically, as has the diversity of the other components of the department community and the patient populations served by the department. The residents are more diverse than the faculty. The medical students are more diverse than the residents. And the patients are more diverse than the students.

Contrasting the four male UMMS-graduate interns who started residency in July 1979, the current thirty-three residents reflect diversity in ways that were inconceivable

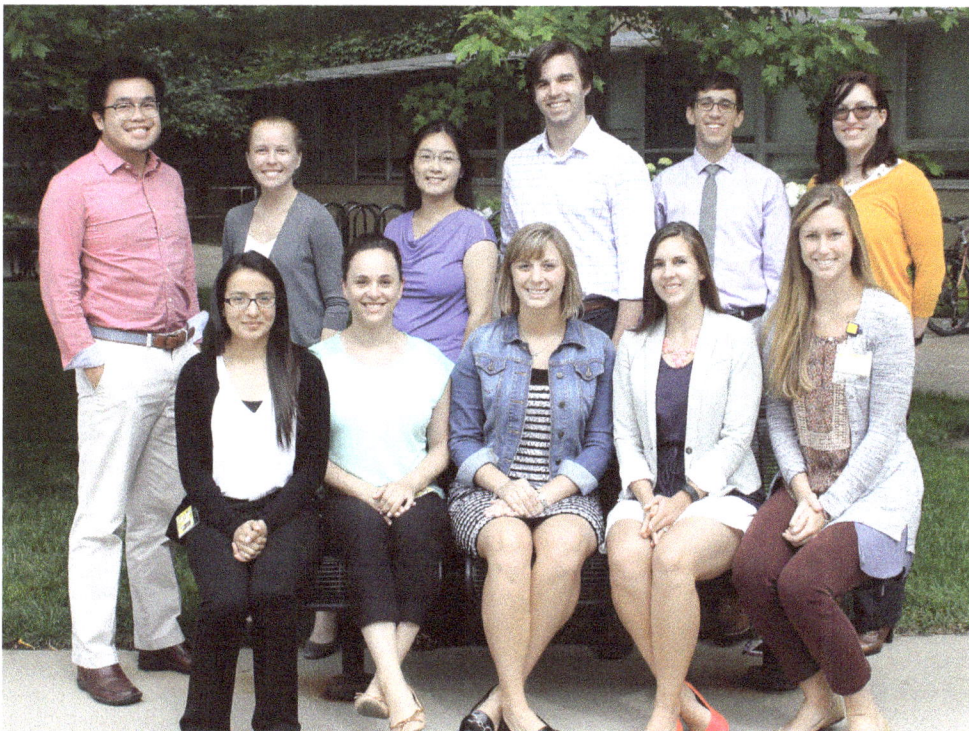

Figure 7.3. Residency class of 2019 (July 2016)

at the outset of the program. Male residents represent 36 percent of the current cohort of residents across classes, and only 15 percent of the current residents are UMMS graduates. There are graduates from twenty-three other medical schools in sixteen states and the District of Columbia among the cohort of thirty-three. There are current residents from two of the allopathic medical schools in the state of Michigan, and a graduate of the MSU College of Osteopathic Medicine was a member of the residency class of 2017, the most recent of many residents who had attended osteopathic medical schools.

Another theme that has become clear in reviewing the history of this department is that some things that happened were simply random or fortuitous. For example, in the interview conducted with Dr. Schwenk in Nevada in January 2016, he reflected upon how important the phone call he received from Dr. Reed indicating her decision to leave Utah and come to Ann Arbor was. At the time, however, it was not clear what direction her husband Dr. Zazove would take his career, such as whether he would pursue options in community practice or as a faculty member.[2] No one could have anticipated the important role he would play in the leadership of the Department of Family Medicine. During an interview in July 2017, Dr. Zazove gave this response when he was asked what he would tell his eventual successor:

Four Suggestions/Lessons Learned
1. Never ever ever ever give up.
2. Focus on getting things done. Success begets success.

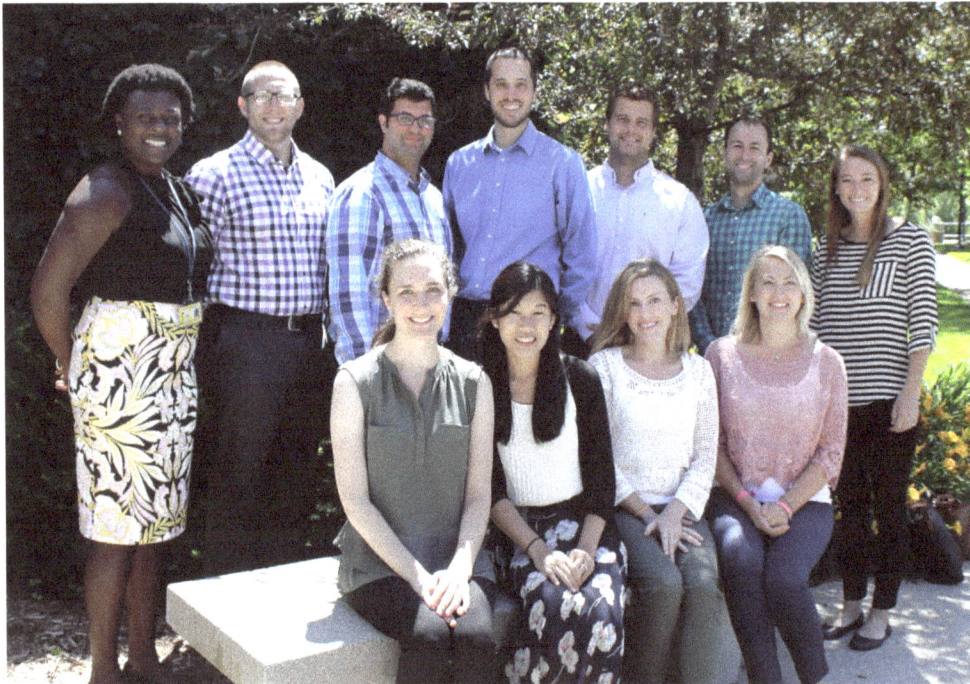

Figure 7.4. Residency class of 2020 (July 2017)

3. Rankings matter.
4. Be visible, be at the table.[3]

While the focus of written documents is on successes and accomplishments, major disappointments and setbacks linger in the memories of those who were present for them. The prolonged uncertainty during the time of the external review process of 1984–85 remains in the forefront of the memories of those who were in the department at that time. The loss of space negotiations and the lack of confidence in family medicine as a viable specialty or discipline are still burrs in the saddles of some longtime department members. Yet these struggles reinforce one of Dr. Zazove's four pieces of advice: "Never ever ever ever give up."

That principle was certainly established even before the department was created. The efforts of local family physicians, alumni, the MAFP, and other groups showed perseverance as they kept knocking on the door of the University of Michigan leadership to get the new specialty of family medicine established. And eventually, with pressure from the state legislature, the door was opened.

Symbolism has remained important in the history of this department. In the early phase, the department was almost entirely Chelsea-centric, for many understandable reasons, but eventually the department needed to move beyond that focus on Chelsea and become more integrated into the larger academic medical center for the department to survive.

The University of Michigan is often described as "a good place to be from." In looking across the history of the University, this adage can be applied both before and after there was a formal Department of Family Medicine. While many future leaders of family practice or medicine went to UMMS long before the department was founded, the establishment of the department and the residency provided more leadership opportunities and brought in faculty, residents, and fellows who would develop into leaders during their time in Ann Arbor. Many of these leaders went on to spread their skills throughout the country. Dr. Davies was the first faculty member to go elsewhere to become chair. After several years on the faculty following completion of his term as chair in 1986, he moved to the Department of Family and Community Medicine at the Eastern Virginia School of Medicine, where he served as professor and chair from 1990 to 2002.

In addition to Dr. Schwenk, another faculty member hired by Dr. Davies went on to become a department chair elsewhere. Ricardo G. Hahn, MD, MS, was a resident at the Medical University of South Carolina (MUSC) when Dr. Davies was on faculty there, and he spent two years at the department in Ann Arbor before moving on to faculty appointments at other medical schools, the last of which was as professor and chair of the University of Southern California Department of Family Medicine. Dr. Hahn was in that position from 1995 to 2006.

More recently, three faculty members have left Ann Arbor to become chairs at other institutions. Lee A. Green, MD, MPH, was named as chair of the Department of Family Medicine at the University of Alberta in 2012. Mack T. Ruffin IV, MD, MPH, left to serve as chair of the Hershey Medical Center Department of Family and Community Medicine at Penn State University in 2016. Grant Greenberg, MD, MHSA, MA, was named chair of the Department of Family Medicine at the Lehigh Valley Health Network in Allentown, Pennsylvania, in 2016. Drs. Green and Greenberg were both graduates of UMMS and the residency program. All three of the faculty members who left had served as an assistant and/or associate chair of one of the key department mission areas.

Another tradition established early on that continues to this day is the celebration of successes. This began with the symposium the Family of Family Medicine, which was conducted in June 1982 in conjunction with the graduation of the first four residents. This tradition has continued with residency graduations and other milestones in the history of the department. More recently the student scholarships and award ceremony has grown in stature in a similar fashion. Starting in 2005 with a small ceremony during grand rounds, it has grown substantially as more scholarships and awards have been added. A luncheon for the scholarship and award honorees and their families was added in 2008. In 2011, a fellowship graduate luncheon was added to the lineup of celebrations.

The celebrations of the founding of the department began with a series of events marking the tenth anniversary in 1988, branded as a "Decade of Caring." Subsequent celebrations have been held in 1998, 2004, 2008, and 2014. April 2018 will mark the fortieth year since the department's founding in 1978 with another celebration.

While the University of Michigan is a "good place to be from" for students, residents, fellows, and faculty members, the department has imported many talented people from elsewhere to serve in key leadership positions. Throughout the history of the department, its continued growth and development have been fueled by recruiting, hiring, and retaining key faculty who had limited or no ties to Ann Arbor or the University prior to coming

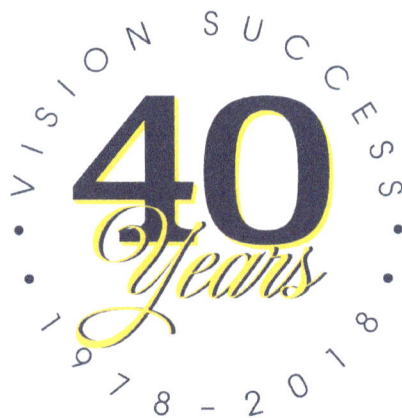

Department of Family Medicine
University of Michigan

as residents or faculty. Later in the timeline, after the establishment of fellowships, fellows also became a new source of faculty and future leaders.

Two of the three chairs were trained exclusively elsewhere, and one left for nine years to complete his family medicine residency and initial community practice and faculty experience before returning in 1984 to become a part of the faculty. All three of the chairs came from places where family medicine was much more established as an academic specialty than it was in the state of Michigan, much less at the University of Michigan. While Dr. Davies came most immediately from the University of South Alabama, his initial academic time in the United States took place at the MUSC, a premier department that attracted residents from all over the country. Coincidentally, Joseph V. Fisher, MD—who had been in practice in Chelsea and was among the proposed directors for the Washtenaw County Family Practice Residency Program that failed to receive accreditation in the early 1970s—took a position as director of behavioral science at the MUSC program and knew Dr. Davies through that connection even before Dr. Davies came to Ann Arbor as the founding chair. Prior to his studies in the United States, Dr. Davies trained and worked in the United Kingdom and Jamaica within a socialized medicine system.

Dr. Schwenk and Dr. Zazove completed their residency training at the University of Utah. Both Dr. Zazove and his wife, Dr. Reed, matched at the University of Utah in the spring of 1978 as Dr. Schwenk was completing his residency at the same program and then starting in community practice in nearby Park City, Utah. While their times there did not overlap directly, they did become acquainted during the years they spent in Utah. When it came time for Dr. Schwenk to recruit Dr. Reed to Ann Arbor as part of his efforts to build up the department's research program, their familiarity with each other and the similar training they had received in Salt Lake City worked to their mutual benefit. Much like MUSC, the Department of Family and Community Medicine at the University of Utah was among the top programs in family medicine at the time. It is interesting to consider what might have happened in March 1978 if Dr. Zazove and Dr. Reed had matched at their first option for residency training, Duke University in Durham, North Carolina, on the other side of the country from Salt Lake City! In this case, getting one's second choice on the couple's match list seems to have turned out well.

All three chairs came from situations and settings that had shown them the family medicine model would work. The challenge was getting the opportunity to try it in Ann Arbor. The foundation and concept of family medicine as an academic discipline was laid by Dr. Davies and then added to and further developed by Drs. Schwenk and Zazove. Those who were hired by Dr. Davies or were students, residents, or fellows during his term can sense that they are all part of a continuum. Similarly, those who entered the story of this department at later points in the timeline can feel their own connections to its development. During their tenures, these three chairs recruited people who advanced one or more department missions. Each recruited or mentored people who became leaders, scholars, innovators, or educators.

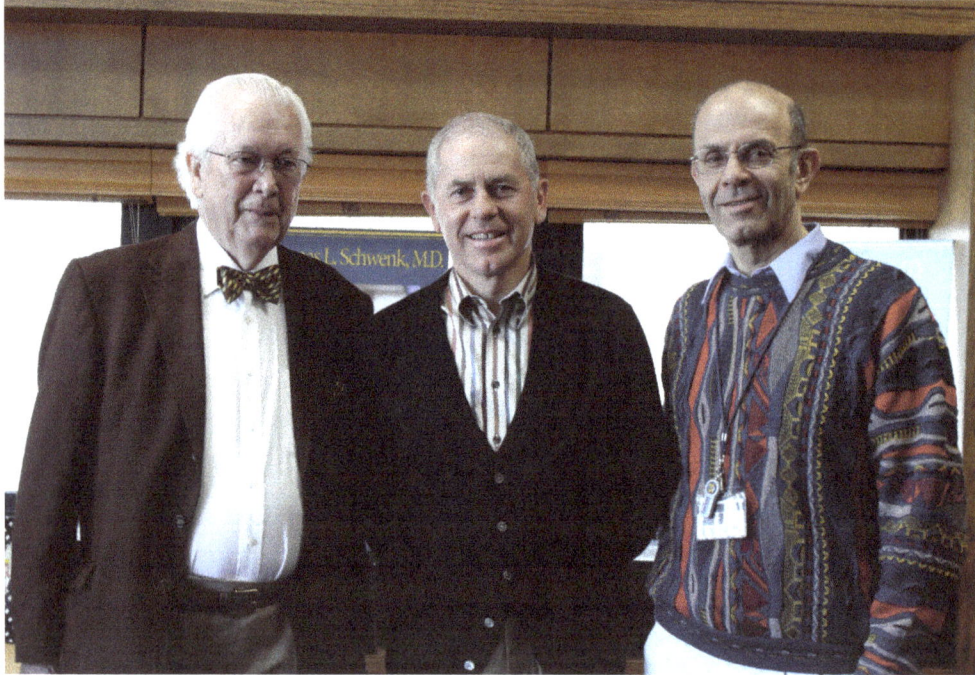

Figure 7.5. We three chairs of Michigan are ... Dr. Davies, Dr. Schwenk, and Dr. Zazove

Another key moment in the maturation of the department was when then Dean Lichter suggested that it expand its development efforts. This fruitful suggestion ultimately led to an increase in scholarships and awards for medical students and residents, two endowed lectureships, and a named chair of family medicine. The incorporation of a development officer and associated activities into the department was another successful move. Compared to development officers at other medical schools, Amy C. St. Amour was fully integrated into the DFM. She had dedicated office space in the department and spent time learning about the specialty and the department's people and programs. On average, in other departments, the length of tenure for someone in that role lasts less than two years, but here she has been the only person in that role since she began in 2003. Additionally, the timing of the hiring of a development officer coincided with a period of success, allowing her to promote the department among alumni—even ones who had been students before the DFM existed—who were now in a position to give back to their alma mater. Many of the people who were part of the initial lobbying to start the department were also able to donate. As is often the case, the department was able to capitalize on the fortunate timing of many factors. As identified in one of Dr. Zazove's four key principles, "success begets success." Over time, more donors have been identified and more scholarships, awards, and bequests have been secured, allowing this success to continue to snowball.

Setbacks and Challenges

Not everything has worked out as planned from day one. This fact seems very easy to appreciate at first glance, but documents, reports, and newsletters often leave out failures and disappointments. While the DFM has had few in comparison with its successes, some examples merit discussion at this time.

Several years ago, one of the chief residents was surprised to learn that years earlier in the department's history, there had been a time when the residency had not filled all its spots through the Match. He was even more shocked when he was told there had been occasions when residents had been dismissed or encouraged to transfer to another program. Again, these are not the kinds of things that are highlighted in residency brochures or during the interview overview session when candidates are in the area for a day, but residents or faculty members who were present during those times would be able to quote examples without much prompting. In a similar fashion, there have been years when UMMS students who applied to family medicine did not match and had to be assisted in the "scramble" process.

The department, as an organization and community, had its share of times when it dealt with severe illnesses, surgeries, and deaths among faculty, residents, fellows, and staff members. These instances tested the resiliency of the collective department community, just as the physicians and others involved in clinical care must be sensitive to the losses among the patient populations served by the department. At the time of the 9/11 attacks, the department chose to hold its State of the Department Address (SODA) and faculty retreat the following day as originally scheduled, despite the fact that the University had canceled classes and other events. The gathering was very therapeutic on that critical day as everyone tried to process the events of the day before and what it would mean. This event was not a topic that showed up in an annual report or newsletter article, but nonetheless it was critical in the department history.

There were other losses or setbacks along the way where individual or community resilience was helpful in properly coping and moving on. Students failed the clerkship, residents failed rotations, and efforts to start new programs were not approved. Notable setbacks included the inability to establish an adolescent medicine fellowship and the failed effort to develop a joint family medicine residency with St. Joseph Mercy Hospital. Yet despite these momentary shortfalls, the department has continued to expand its involvement in the care of adolescent patients in the region. Even though the DFM was not able to expand the size of the residency by combining efforts with St. Joseph Mercy in the past, the entering class of interns will increase in number from eleven to thirteen as a result of other developments since that time. In both these cases, the initial efforts did not work out as planned, but in the long run, the ultimate goals were met through different channels. Just as small businesses must adjust to losses and setbacks, the department had to do likewise and keep moving forward.

Themes across Chairs

Two key areas that have not been specifically highlighted in previous chapters are faculty development and continuing medical education (CME). From the very beginning, both of these areas were high on the agenda dating back to the July 1978 planning priorities list created by Dr. Davies. Via a combination of resources, the three chairs were able to provide support for faculty to develop their baseline of knowledge and skills in areas related to patient care, teaching, administration, scholarly writing, and research. Over time, many of the people who participated in local or national faculty development programs were able to use those skills to teach other faculty or fellows through a "train the trainer" model. And because the department also had opportunities for faculty to both direct and teach in CME programs, there were other opportunities for them to apply the skills in ways beyond teaching students and residents.

The three chairs used some outstanding local, regional and national options for further education. The presence of an excellent School of Public Health (SPH) created opportunities for junior faculty with aspirations of academic careers to participate in what was then called the On-Job-On-Campus (OJOC) program, a series of intense educational coursework that could lead to a master's degree in one of several departments within the SPH. Several of the first faculty to participate in OJOC went on to become leaders of the DFM's research programs.

Along with OJOC, the department sponsored faculty to participate in the MSU Primary Care Faculty Development Fellowship Program. This program was less intense than OJOC and did not lead to a master's degree, but it did require spending time in East Lansing, which took people away from patient care and teaching obligations for several weeks across the term of the fellowship. Another benefit of the MSU and OJOC programs was that participants came from around the country and from other medical specialties and health care professions. Both these programs exposed participants to faculty from other parts of the country and other disciplines, which often led to future research and educational collaborations.

As mentioned previously, the department was successful from early on in getting training grants funded by the Division of Medicine. An outcome of one of the funded training grants was the establishment of the University of Michigan Family Medicine Faculty Development Institute (FDI), which continues to this day in a condensed version of its original format. Dr. Sheets has served as the director of the FDI since it began in July 1994. The FDI requires less of a time commitment than the OJOC or the MSU programs but fills a niche in terms of providing at least thirty hours of teaching that is focused on core skills in classroom and clinical teaching, assessment of learners, curriculum development and management, and administrative skills.

Another program with a long tradition was established within the medical school with the advent of the Medical Education Scholars Program (MESP) in 1997. While the FDI was a series of whole-day sessions conducted off campus in a local hotel, the MESP was a series of thirty to thirty-six afternoon sessions conducted on campus, administered by another medical school department. A number of department faculty participated in the MESP, often after completing the FDI. Currently, the academic fellow also participates in the MESP. Similar to the MSU fellowship and OJOC program, MESP provides a chance for junior faculty and fellows to meet people from other departments in the medical school.

There was also a tradition established early on to support faculty who needed to go elsewhere to gain skills in procedural training or specific research training. Three prime examples involved sending faculty to get training in colposcopy, obstetrical ultrasonography, and evidence-based medicine.

There is some overlap between faculty development and CME. The major difference is that before the department existed, there were some CME courses run by the UMMS that were geared at general practitioners and family physicians. Eventually, the department took over leadership of these courses from a medical school department that had administered all CME courses. In addition to the traditional review course held in Ann Arbor, there were summer and winter CME programs, both held in northern Michigan at ski or golf resorts. Later, for a number of years, there was a procedures course held on campus and a women's health course run in conjunction with the Department of Obstetrics and Gynecology and a Sports Medicine course. Over the years, some of the economics of conducting CME courses changed, and the department cut back on the number of course offerings. The DFM has gone through several models for administering these courses. Regardless of the model of administration or the focus of topics for these CME courses, they have continued to be favorably evaluated by participants and continue to be a core component of the department's educational programs.

The department has had a unique experience working with members of the local Deaf and hard-of-hearing community thanks to Dr. Zazove. He has developed a strong following in the local area, particularly at his practice site in Dexter. He has published extensively in this area and given numerous grand rounds and medical student presentations, often while including patients and sign language interpreters.

Over time, each clinical site has developed ways in which it has been able to serve unique segments of the communities in which it is located. Early on in the development of the Chelsea practice, sports physicals for middle and high school students were offered as a service and a way to market the practice to the community. The practice sponsored fun runs and a booth at the Chelsea Community Fair. As additional practices were added, each found relevant ways to get incorporated into the communities it served.

The DFM has responded to opportunities to expand into different areas of clinical service over the years. One clinical service area that cut across sites and settings was sports medicine. For a period of several years, members of the department served as team doctors to high school football teams across Washtenaw County. Later, as the sports medicine fellowship developed ties at Eastern Michigan and the University of Michigan, faculty and fellows began serving in key roles in the care of women's and men's athletes at both institutions, a tradition that continues to date.

The DFM had an early connection to the Corner Health Center in Ypsilanti, which continues to serve adolescent patients in the area. In more recent years, the department

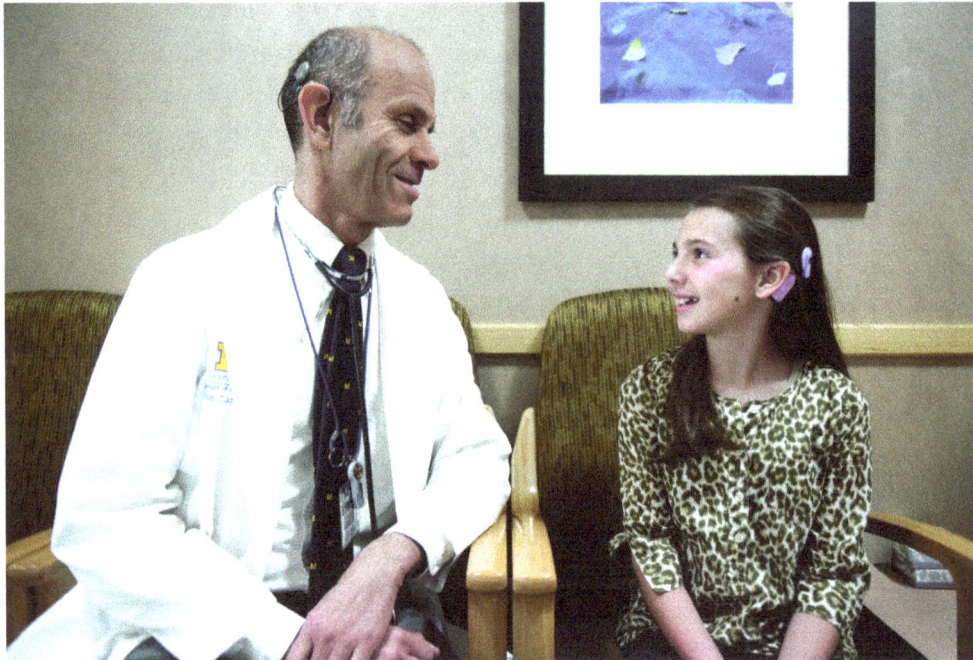

Figure 7.6. Dr. Zazove and a patient

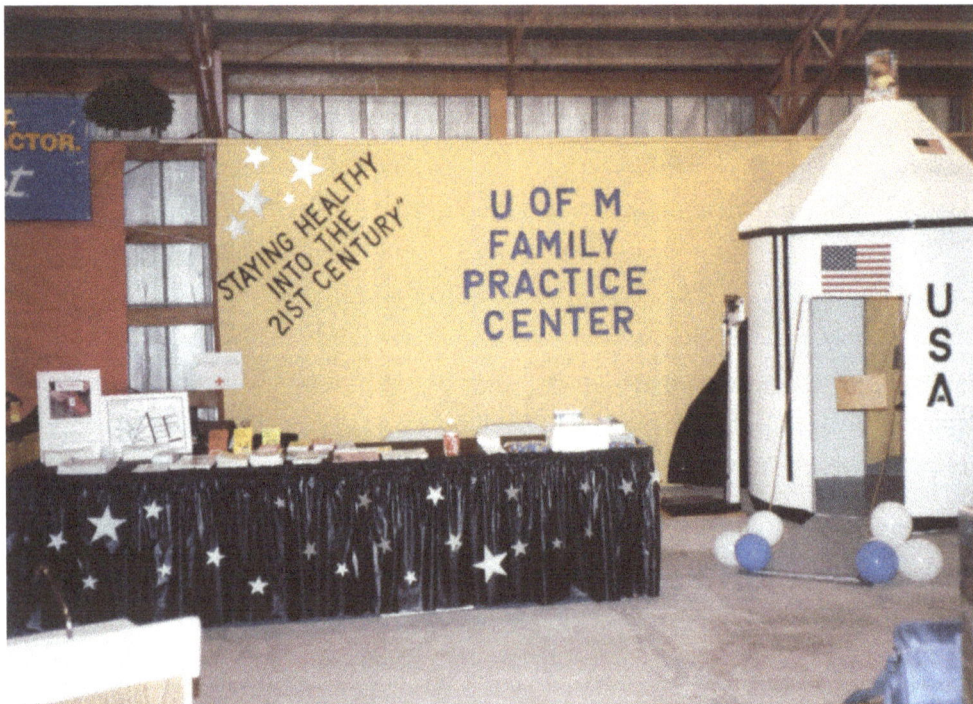

Figure 7.7. Chelsea Community Fair booth

has provided physician coverage within a collaborative effort across multiple middle schools and high schools in the region. While the adolescent fellowship was never established as hoped, the department's role in caring for adolescent populations has been a strong interest that has endured.

Care of the medically underserved has been another recurrent focus of those in the department. Involvement in migrant clinics and other free clinics has been linked with student and resident education whenever possible.

Individual faculty members have pursued international experiences, sometimes on their own and sometimes through department-sponsored initiatives, most notably in Japan and Ghana. Faculty and learners of all levels have also come from these two countries in particular to spend time in the department.

Legends, Lore, and Legacy

Comments made by those involved in the story of this department are helpful for providing context to certain issues. One question that sometimes arises at national meetings is why the department was named the Department of Family Practice rather than Department of Family Medicine prior to 1997. Department lore provides the answer. Though unsubstantiated, it is claimed that someone with great influence in the school and health system said at the time of the establishment of the department: "As long as I am here, the only department of medicine at the University of Michigan will be the Department of Internal Medicine." By the time of the second department review in 1996, when external consultants recommended that the department be renamed the Department of Family Medicine, it just so happened that the person who was reported to have made the comment in 1978 was no longer in Ann Arbor.

The previous anecdote regarding the name change of the department has a corollary. Others outside the department would sometimes shorten the name of the specialty to "family." This quirk was first noticed when medical students were overheard talking about what rotation they were on or what specialty they were considering pursuing and they would say "family" instead of "family medicine." And thus it became part of the nomenclature of the environment, just as "pediatrics" has long been shortened to "peds," "orthopedic surgery" to "ortho," and so on. The adoption of an abbreviated term of reference was another sign of the gradual acceptance and incorporation of family medicine into the culture of the University.

Another critical decision made by Dr. Davies in 1978 was to hire a PhD educator as the first faculty member rather than someone with a medical degree. Certainly this was out-of-the-box thinking at the time in Ann Arbor, and there was push back from others in the medical school administration at the thought of a clinical department hiring a faculty member with a PhD in higher education administration, but Dr. Davies persevered and hired the first of many faculty members without medical degrees who were to play major roles in the evolution in the department across all missions and functions. At the outset, student education, residency education, continuing medical education, faculty development, and department administration were the primary activities for Dr. Lefever and others with degrees outside medicine. Over time, the role of faculty and staff with other graduate degrees has become equally critical to the success of research and clinical programs. This practice eventually has come to be more prevalent in other areas of the medical center and clinical departments.

A number of stories contribute to the legends, lore, and legacy over the years. As described previously, the external review of 1984 lingered on for an inordinately long time, causing unsubstantiated rumors in the community about the department shutting down or being made into a division of the Department of Internal Medicine. One of the little known moments of that time occurred when the interim dean Peter A. Ward, MD, independently called two faculty members in to meet with him in his office. Dean Ward met with both Dr. O'Brien and Dr. Peggs independently and without their knowledge of his meeting with the other. During these meetings, both were assured that if the department was dissolved or made into a division of another department, their faculty positions and clinical practice would be maintained. At some point over the years, after the department had been maintained as a full department, the legend grew that one of the issues that came up in those independent meetings was that the University wanted to maintain a presence in Chelsea in order to help protect the western edge of the clinical enterprise from any excursions from the north and west by MSU. As the story was retold over the years, it became a myth that the medical center was worried about an incursion by "green and white hordes" of Spartans swooping down from the north and west. While this was clearly not the specific content of the conversation between the interim dean and two family physician faculty members, it is an example of how sometimes a kernel of truth can be expanded over time.

Inside the department, there has been a long tradition of referring to the "family of family medicine," dating back to that first major symposium in June 1982. When there was a coed softball team started by the residents and continued by the faculty for several years in the mid to late 1980s, the team was officially listed in the softball league schedule as "Chelsea Family." This led one coach of another team to ask one of the players if the rumor was true that the majority of the players were from a large family in Chelsea. Another time, when a player on a nearby softball diamond was injured sliding into a base in the era before omnipresent cell phones, someone came over to where Chelsea Family was playing and asked if it was true that some of the team members were doctors, and if so, could someone come look at the injured player before they called 911?

From the very beginning, the DFM was also a family in the sense that S. Margaret Davies, MD, was one of the first faculty members and developed her own role and visibility within the department and medical school beyond being married to the first chair. One way she got involved was by joining the Medical School Admissions Committee. In that role, she also became involved with the Galens Medical Society and subsequently

> ### Comments from "Building on a Vision" Document from 1998 Anniversary Celebration: Building a Community
>
> "We had a real spirit of camaraderie at Chelsea. Sometimes we'd close early on a Friday afternoon and have a little party. We played softball games and I remember us getting into a big argument with an opposing team, a bunch of lawyers."[4]
>
> *James F. Peggs, MD*

served as an unofficial adviser to many students regardless of specialty interest. Being based off-site in Chelsea likely facilitated the chance that students would seek her out for guidance without working through official medical school channels.

This contact eventually led Dr. M. Davies to be portrayed by a medical student as the lead of the 1985 Galens Smoker, an annual student-run comedy performance. That year's production of "Merry Poopins" included a scene where the character of Maggie Poopins descended from the ceiling of the Michigan Theater stage on a commode with an umbrella. Several members of the cast and crew not only followed Dr. M. Davies into the specialty of family medicine, but several have gone on into leadership roles of great importance in other specialties throughout the medical center.

Space and Setting Challenges

Another challenge shared by all the chairs has been securing and retaining appropriate space for clinical, administrative, educational, and research purposes. That challenge has played out time and time again since 1978 and will continue to be a critical issue as the department moves to new space yet again in the coming months. Along with space, a corresponding issue has been finding a way to make the department much less Chelsea-centric. Primary among the reasons for this has been the logistics of getting people together in person for grand rounds and other conferences and faculty meetings and resident conferences. As the department spread to the east from Chelsea into Ann Arbor and Ypsilanti, there was a need for more centralized space, especially as the department outgrew the available space in Chelsea. Space was rented off campus for a while at the Environmental Research Institute of Michigan (ERIM) before moving to the new East Ann Arbor Health Center when it opened on Plymouth Road in 1996. Following the move of the administrative offices to Women's Hospital in 1999, the department shifted large group presentations and faculty meetings to Ford Auditorium in the University Hospital and resident conferences and other meetings to conference room space at Women's. With the upcoming move to the 300 North Ingalls building, which will distance the administrative offices even more from the center of the medical center, new logistical challenges associated with convening for educational programs and meetings will need to be addressed.

In looking over various sources in compiling this department history, it becomes clear from a somewhat subjective perspective that this is a unique department in a special setting. While it would be presumptuous to conclude that it is one of a kind, that assessment might be not too far off the mark! One of the candidates for the most recent chair search made comments to the effect that he had been a faculty member in two settings at that point in his career in 2012. He had been a faculty member in a top-ten family medicine department at a less prestigious medical school and university, where the family medicine department was much higher rated than either the school or the institution. Then he moved to a very prestigious medical school where he was the founding chair in the same fashion as Dr. Davies in 1978. One reason for his interest in interviewing for the chair position in Ann Arbor was to explore what it was like in a top-ten family medicine department at a top-ten school and institution, in essence combining the characteristics of his previous and current positions. The sentiment that the University of Michigan Department of Family Medicine is unique in its success in such a competitive and challenging environment is shared throughout the community of academic family medicine. The challenge moving forward will be to keep the DFM in this lofty position among its peers.

It is important to try to identify what makes a department like this one special, or "Not Just Any Department of Family Medicine" functioning inside "Not Just Any Medical School." As with any organization, success starts with the leadership, and the DFM has been blessed with visionary leaders from the outset. The initial support from local family physicians and state and national academies and the pressure from the Michigan State Legislature all led to the beginning of this adventure in March 1978. Along the way, the establishment of family medicine in such a research-oriented tertiary care setting has had its highs and lows, but when there were opportunities to succeed and supportive leadership, the department was able to "step up to the plate" and be successful. None of this would have been possible without the involvement of talented and committed people. In considering the traits of the people, programs, and services provided by this department since 1978, here are the characteristics that came to mind:

Loyalty
Productivity
Competence
Continuity
Creativity
Vision
Compassion
Planning
Preparedness
Adaptability
Perseverance

The department has cared for tens of thousands of patients over the years. One patient wrote a letter dated September 8, 2017, which was read at the 2017 SODA by Elizabeth K. Jones, MD, the medical director at the Livonia Health Center where the patient received care. The sentiments are likely shared by patients from all of the department's sites in reference to multiple faculty, fellows, residents, and staff since 1978.

I am writing to tell you how impressed I am, as a patient, with the level of care I have received at the Livonia Health Center.

I feel like the Livonia Health Center exemplifies the best not only in family medicine, but the best in Michigan health care. First, the support staff, the people who answer the phones, greet patients, and keep the office humming are the most professional I have met in my multiple visits to clinics within the U of M system. They are always polite to me, and to others, and seem to take care of each person who walks in as if that person were a member of their family. More so, they speak in quiet tones, maintain confidentiality, and really seem to do their best to make patients feel comfortable. The fact that these individuals are able to maintain a stable and professional demeanor is commendable.

Thank you for all the hard work at this clinic. I realize family medicine may not be the most glamorous of specialties, but I wanted you to know how much an exemplary family medicine clinic, with good staff and providers, can mean to one patient. So, thank you.[5]

In addition to the words of that patient, students have summed up why the department has been successful in its various mission areas for forty years. Vikas K. Jayadeva, recipient of the 2017 Paddy and Donald N. Fitch, MD, Scholarship and the 2016–17 Harold Kessler, MD, Family Medicine Scholarship, stated, "My decision to become a family physician comes from an understanding of the mechanisms of disease but even more so from dealing with the personal and social aspects of the ailment. To me, this means working across medical specialties to prevent illness, rather than reacting to it. It also means holistically addressing the health care inequalities that ignited my passion for medicine. But the most compelling aspects of family medicine for me are the longitudinal patient relationships that are developed, nurtured and maintained, forming the cornerstone of excellent patient management."[6] Elizabeth M. Irish, recipient of the 2016 Michael Papo, MD, Scholarship, shared, "As someone who enjoys intellectual challenges, understanding people in their unique context, and working hard for those who place their trust in you, a career in family medicine is wholly encompassing for me. These principles, along with those that I will learn as I continue training, are not just valuable lessons learned from my medical education, but are the guiding principles that I will use in the care of my future patients and their loved ones as a family physician."[7]

With testimonials from patients and students like these, the future continues to be bright for the University of Michigan Department of Family Medicine. Dr. Zazove summarized the 2016 Scholarship and Awards Event in this fashion: "It was so stimulating to see these scholarships being presented to the fourth-year students headed to family medicine residencies across the country. Hearing stories of the incredible accomplishments of these students as well as the background of the donors was inspiring. It is clear that family medicine will be in good hands with the next generation."[8]

In reviewing documents and reports written across the last forty years, reading emails and letters, and listening to interviews with key historical figures, it was readily evident how important the "family of family medicine" has been in establishing this department from day one. This legacy has continued across the terms of three chairs, all of whom came from different places and backgrounds but found common themes, challenges, and successes in an environment that was not always fully supportive or appreciative of what they were trying to accomplish.

In his final column in a spring 2011 newsletter, Dr. Schwenk summarized the department's accomplishments: "I believe we have created something truly special in Family Medicine at U-M. And I am not using the royal 'we' (as I sometimes do). I really mean 'we.' The Department's growth and development has been more of a crusade than a job, a crusade that was fueled by the commitment and energy of every single member of the Department. We have established Family Medicine as a major contributor to and source of pride by the University of Michigan Health System, something many people said could not be done in our early years."[9]

In the six years since Dr. Schwenk wrote that closing column after his twenty-five years of serving as chair, the department has continued to pursue that crusade under the leadership of Dr. Zazove. He has built upon the foundation established by Drs. Davies and Schwenk with the assistance of countless faculty colleagues, fellows, residents, students, staff members, and friends who have supported the department and its commitment to excellence across its mission areas of patient care, education, research, and service.

A cumulative timeline of key events and individuals in department history follows this closing chapter along with notes and sources used in documenting the accomplishments, stories, and anecdotes shared throughout this book. The appendices provide lists of key members of the "family of family medicine" at the University of Michigan dating back to March 1, 1978, as well as recognizing those individuals who have received awards or scholarships based on their academic, teaching, clinical, research, service, and scholarly accomplishments. Lastly, the friends and supporters of the department who have provided gifts and donations in support of programs, scholarships, and awards are acknowledged in grateful appreciation for their past, present, and future support.

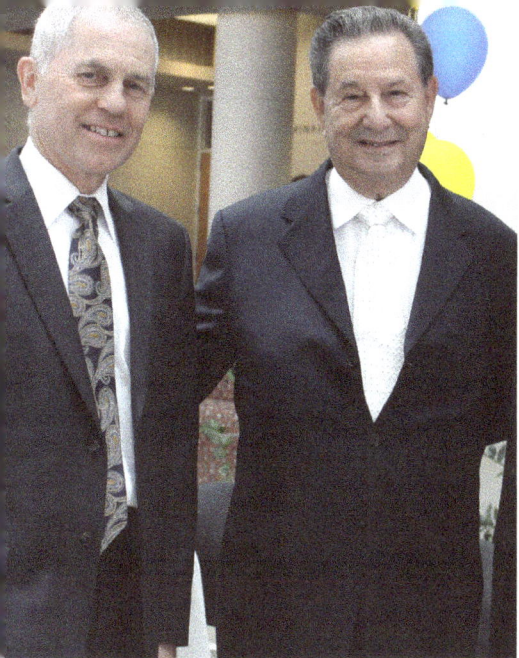

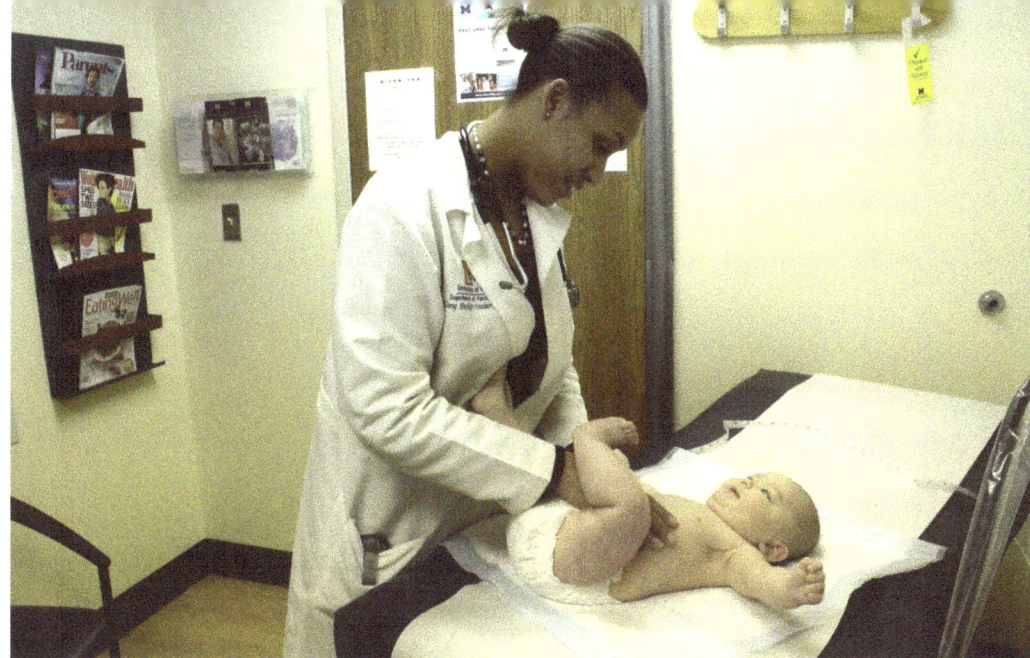

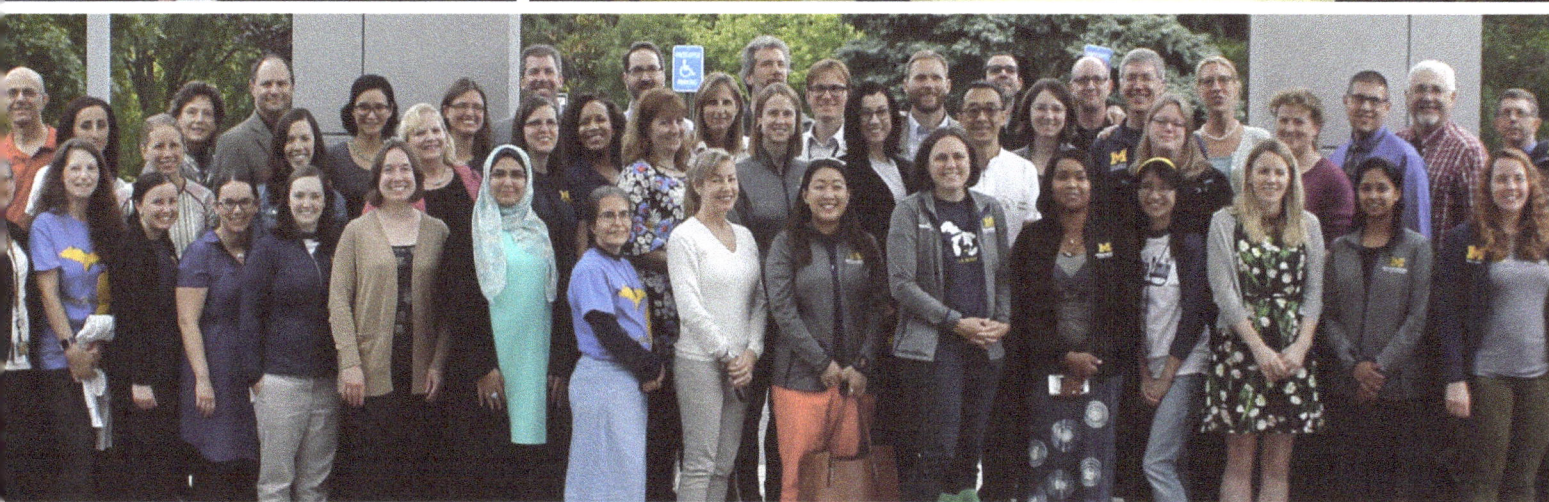

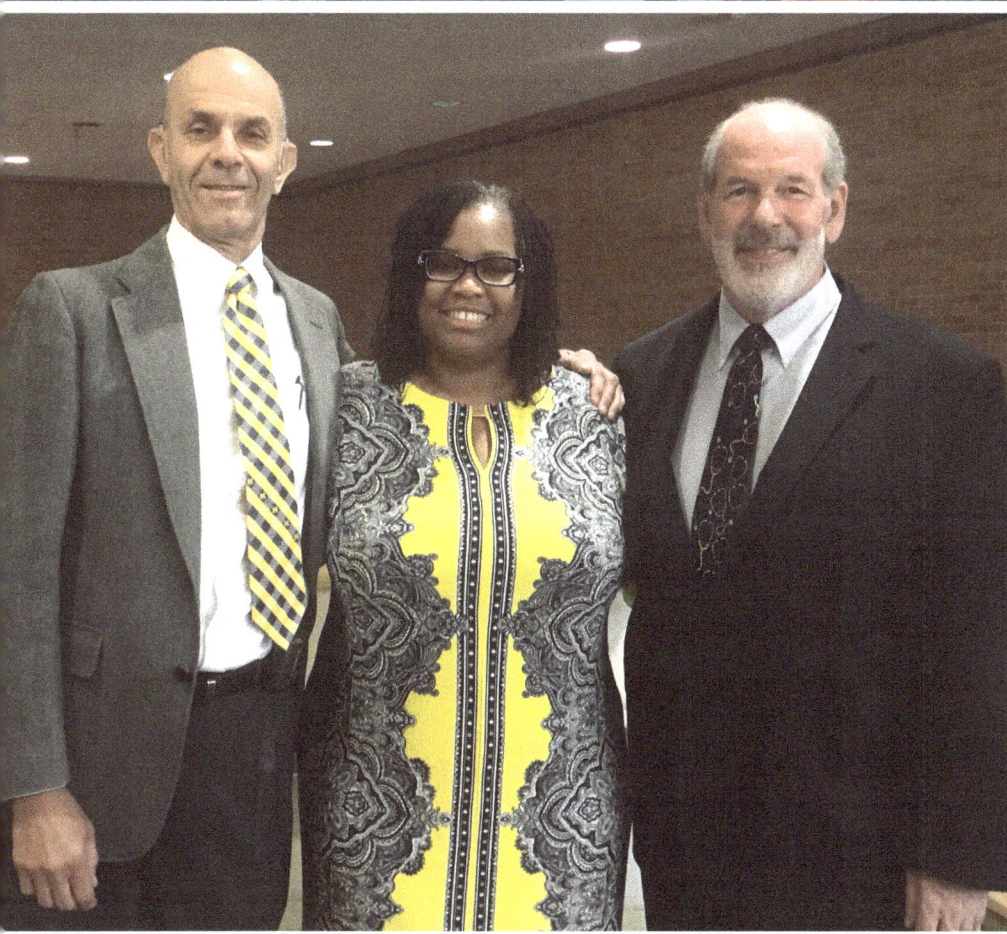

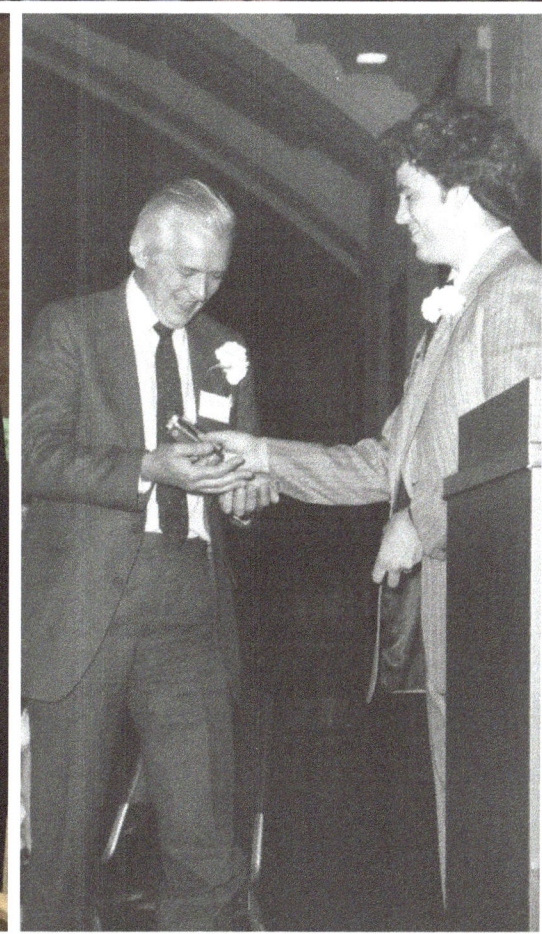

THE
UNIVERSITY OF
MICHIGAN
FAMILY PRACTICE
CENTER

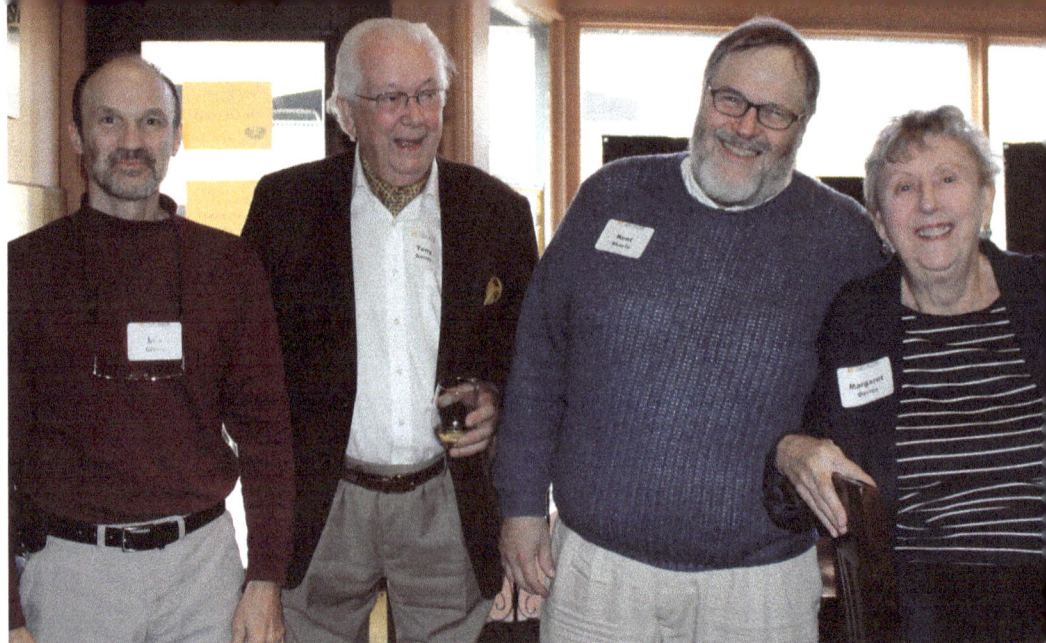

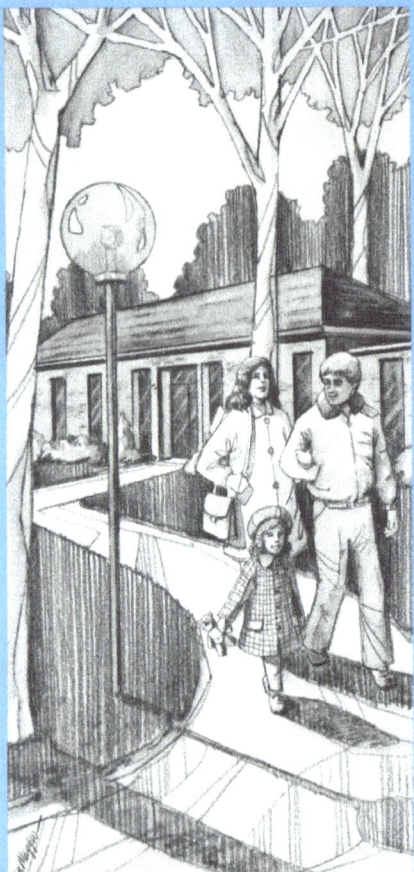

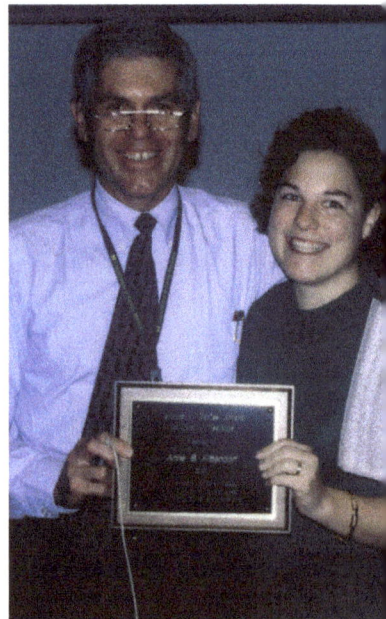

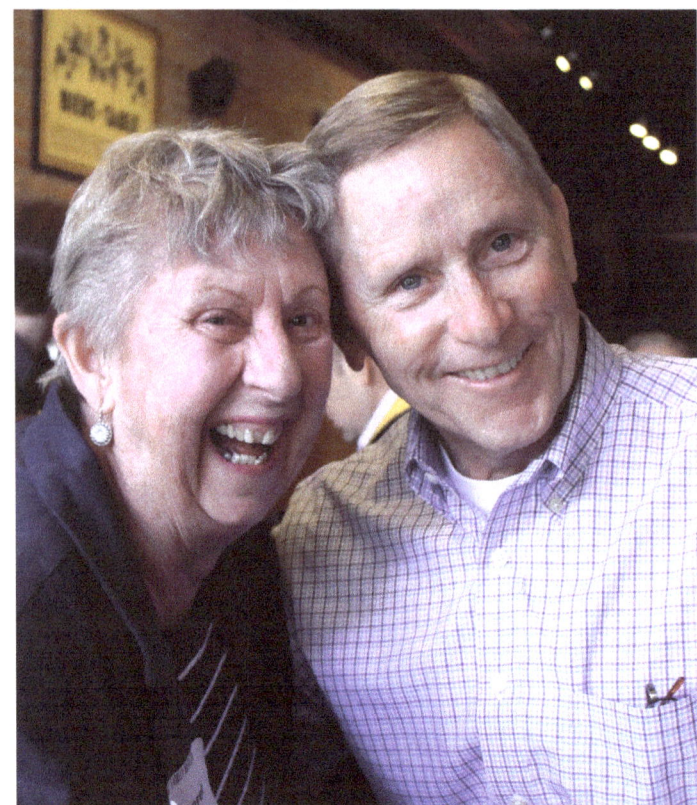

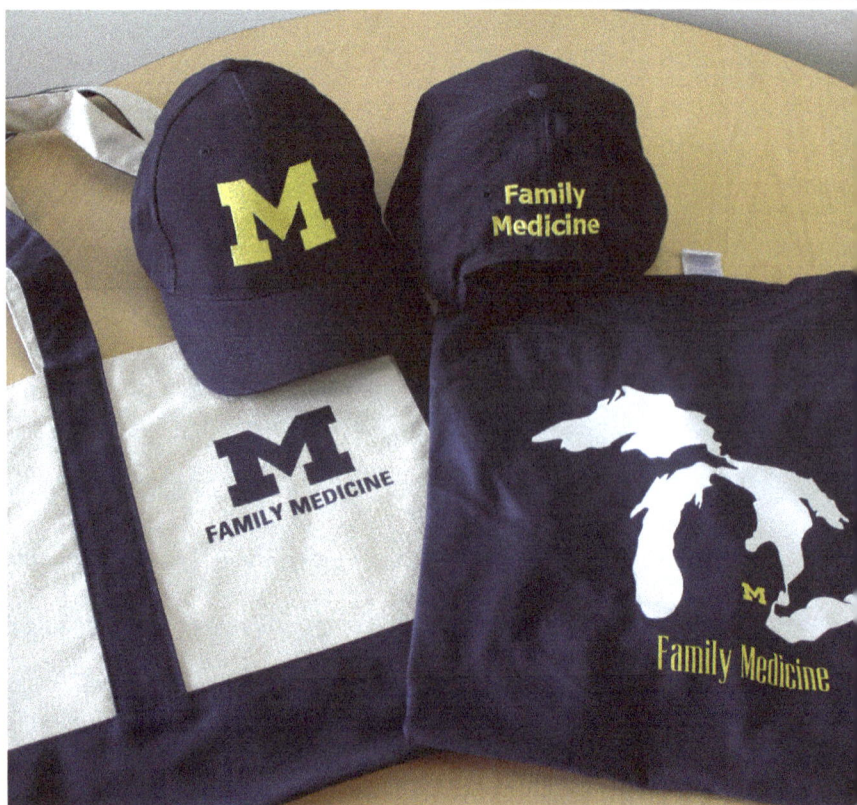

Cumulative Timeline
1966 to 2017

Chapter 1 Timeline: Key Events/Individuals between 1966 and 1978

1966	American Medical Association releases national reports: Millis Commission Report and Willard Report
1967	Society of Teachers of Family Medicine (STFM) is established
1969	American Board of Family Practice is established
1971	American Academy of General Practice changes to American Academy of Family Physicians (AAFP)
1971	Michigan State Legislature resolutions to establish departments of family practice at the three state university allopathic medical schools
1972–73	Washtenaw County family practice residency proposal is submitted and denied
February 1975	Michigan Academy of Family Physicians (MAFP) representatives meet with Board of Regents and Dean Gronvall
October 1975	Residency planning committee is established
November 1976	Board of Regents approves Department of Family Practice
January 1977	AAFP and Ostergaard Consultation Report recommends Chelsea as clinical site
October 1977	Terence C. Davies, MD, accepts offer to serve as first chair

Chapter 2 Timeline: Key Events/Individuals between 1978 and 1986

March 1, 1978	First day of the department
1978	First residency director appointed: R. Dale Lefever, PhD
1978	First service chief: Dr. Davies
1979	Accreditation and residency training grant is approved
July 1979	Entry of first class of four residents

1981	Move to Clinical Faculty Office Building
June 17–18, 1982	Family in Family Medicine Symposium
June 30, 1982	Graduation of first four residents
1983	First assistant chair: Dr. Lefever
1983 to 1984	Internal review process
1984	Move to 1018 Fuller
September 1984	Thomas L. Schwenk, MD, joins faculty
1984	Second residency director: Dr. Schwenk
1984–85	External review process
1985	First newsletter edition
March 1, 1986	Dr. Schwenk begins term as interim chair

Chapter 3 Timeline: Key Events/Individuals between 1986 and 1996

October 1986	First SODA (State of Department Address)
1986	Third residency director: John M. O'Brien, MD
1986	Second service chief: Dr. Schwenk
December 1986	Opening of the first Briarwood site
April 1987	Newborn Privileges Document
March 1988	"Decade of Caring" celebration
May 1988	Delineation of pediatric admitting privileges
June 1988	First student award: Terence C. Davies, MD, award
1988–89	Initiation of University Family Practice (UFP) service
1988–89	First family physician geriatric fellow: David R. Mehr, MD, MS
September 1, 1988	Dr. Schwenk begins term as second chair
October 1989	First faculty retreat
September 1989	Philip Zazove, MD, joins faculty
September 1990	First full-time department administrator: Francine M. Bomar
1991	First associate chair: James F. Peggs, MD
1992	First sports medicine fellow: Robert B. Kiningham, MD, MA
1993	Purchase of Edmunds and Fisher practice in Ypsilanti
1994	Opening of Northeast Ann Arbor site on Green Road
1994	Family practice and obstetrics consultation and privileges guidelines
1995	Reorganization of department leadership structure

1995	First assistant chair of education: Dr. Peggs
1995	First assistant chair of research: Barbara D. Reed, MD, MSPH
1995	First assistant chair of clinical programs: Dr. Zazove
1995	Opening of new Chelsea Health Center
1995	Expansion of residency to Ypsilanti
1995	Establishment of the Japanese Family Health Program
1996	First clerkship director: Dr. Peggs
1996	Opening of Ypsilanti Health Center
1996	Purchase of Dexter Village Family Physicians
1996	Opening of East Ann Arbor Health Center site on Plymouth Road

Chapter 4 Timeline: Key Events/Individuals between 1996 and 2001

July 1996	Beginning of M3 required clerkship
1996	Opening of Ypsilanti Health Center
1996	Second department review
1997	Department name is changed to Department of Family Medicine
February 1997	Move to second Briarwood site
1997	Initiation of educational relative value unit (RVU) system
1997	Opening of Livonia Health Center
1997	Second assistant chair of research: Lee A. Green, MD, MPH
1997	Second assistant chair of clinical programs: Raymond R. Rion, MD
May 1998	Twenty year celebration event, "Building on a Vision"
1998	Opening of Dexter Health Center
1998	Hundredth resident graduates
1998	Opening of Stockbridge Health Center
1999	Establishment of Complementary and Alternative Medicine Research Center
February 1999	Establishment of University Family Medicine (UFM) inpatient service
May 1999	Move of administrative offices to Women's Hospital
1999	First National Institutes of Health (NIH) funding ranking among family medicine departments: third place
1999	Dr. Peggs is named MAFP Family Medicine Educator of the Year
January 2000	Closure of Beyer Hospital

2000	Closure of Stockbridge Health Center
2000	Closure of Livonia Health Center
2000	First University of Michigan Medical School female faculty member is promoted to rank of clinical professor: Barbara S. Apgar, MD, MS
2001	Third internal review process

Chapter 5 Timeline: Key Events/Individuals between 2001 and 2011

July 2001	UFP is renamed Family Mother Baby (FMB) Service
2001	Appointment of Eric P. Skye, MD, as vice-chief of medicine service, Chelsea Community Hospital
2002	Fourth residency director: Dr. Skye
2002	Third assistant chair of clinical programs: Jean M. Malouin, MD, MPH
2002	Dr. Schwenk is elected to the Institute of Medicine
2002	First *US News and World Report* (*USNWR*) department ranking: eighth place
2003	First development officer: Amy C. St. Amour
2003	Michael L. Szymanski, MD, is named MAFP Michigan Family Physician of the Year
2003	Dr. Schwenk receives Society of Teachers of Family Medicine (STFM) Recognition Award
2004	Third assistant chair of research: Mack T. Ruffin IV, MD, MPH
2004	Initiation of Department of Family Medicine Senior Scholarship
2004	ClinfoTracker is licensed
2004	Twenty-five-year anniversary event
2005	First scholarship and awards event
2005	Initiation of William Clippert Gorenflo Research Award in Family Medicine
2005	Initiation of Harold Kessler, MD, Scholarship in Family Medicine
2005	Initiation of Kenneth and Judy Betz Family Medicine Scholarship
2005	Initiation of development advisory committee
2005	Second department administrator: Quinta Vreede
2005	Dr. O'Brien is named MAFP Family Medicine Educator of the Year
2006	First assistant chair of information management and quality: Dr. Green
2006	First academic fellow: Jill N. Fenske, MD

2006	East Ann Arbor Health Center site is relocated to Domino's Farms
June 2007	First George A. Dean, MD, Chair of Family Medicine: Dr. Schwenk
2007	Opening of Latino health clinic at Ypsilanti Health Center
2007	First emeritus faculty member: Dr. Lefever
2007	Second clerkship director: Joel J. Heidelbaugh, MD
2007	Fifth residency director: James M. Cooke, MD
2007	Second assistant chair of education: Dr. Skye
2007	Dr. Peggs named assistant dean for student programs
2007	Assistant chairs are redesignated as associate chairs
2007	First senior associate chair: Dr. Peggs
2007	Dr. Skye is named MAFP Family Medicine Educator of the Year
2007	First Integrative Medicine Fellow: Andrew H. Heyman, MD, MHSA
2008	First scholarship and awards luncheon
2008	Thirty-year-anniversary event
2008	First Hospice and Palliative Medicine Fellow: J. Brandon Walters, MD
2008	Dr. Sheets receives STFM Excellence in Education Award
2008	Election of Dr. Skye as chief of staff, Chelsea Community Hospital
2009	Initiation of collaboration with Ghana College of Physicians and Surgeons
2009	Initiation of Dale L. Williams, MD, Family Medicine Scholarship
2009	Initiation of Vincent P. and Genevieve L. Burns Family Medicine Scholarship
2009	Initiation of Chelsea Community Family Medicine Scholarship
2009	Initiation of Jill and Thomas R. Berglund, MD, Family Medicine Scholarship
2009	First Women's Health Fellow: Ebony C. Parker-Featherstone, MD
2010	Initiation of Alpha Epsilon Iota (AEI) Sorority Family Medicine Scholarship
2010	Third department administrator: Matthew Bazzani
2010	Third service chief: William E. Chavey II, MD
2010	Blythe A. Bieber is selected as recipient of University of Michigan's Health System Support Staff of the Year Award
2010	Initiation of Summer Preceptorship Program
2011	Initiation of Robert J. Fisher, MD, Family Medicine Scholarship

Chapter 6 Timeline: Key Events/Individuals between 2011 and 2017

2011	Dr. Schwenk accepts position at the University of Nevada
2011	Dr. Zazove is named interim chair
2011	First Dr. Max and Buena Lichter Research Professor of Family Medicine: Dr. Ruffin
2012	Second associate chair for information management and quality: Grant M. Greenberg, MD, MSHA, MA
2012	Stefani A. Hudson, MD, is named MAFP Michigan Family Physician of the Year
2012	Dr. Cooke is named executive director of University of Michigan Health System (UMHS) Clinical Simulation Center
2012	Dr. Peggs is inducted into inaugural class of UMMS League of Clinical Excellence
2012	Dr. Reed receives Physician Mentorship Recognition Award from the American Medical Association Women Physicians Congress
2012	Initiation of Paddy and Donald N. Fitch, MD, Family Medicine Scholarship
August 2012	Implementation of MiChart, outpatient electronic medical record
2012	Dr. Zazove is appointed third department chair and second George A. Dean, MD, chair
May 2013	Move from women's to the Medical Science I seventh-floor suite
2013	Sixth residency director: Margaret L. Dobson, MD
2013	Fourth associate chair of clinical programs: David C. Serlin, MD
2013	Sara L. Warber, MD, is awarded Fulbright Scholarship
2013	Drs. Cooke, Peggs, Sheets, and Skye are inducted into inaugural class of UMMS League of Educational Excellence
2013	Dr. Peggs is awarded the MAFP Archie Award of Excellence
2013	Kathrine J. Gold, MD, MSW, MS, is selected as the James C. Puffer, MD/ American Board of Family Medicine fellow at the National Academy of Medicine
2013	Randall T. Forsch, MD, MPH, is named chief medical officer of Chelsea Community Hospital
April 2014	Thirty-five-year anniversary event
2014	Initiation of Terence C. Davies, MD, Endowed Lectureship in Medical Education
2014	Dr. Sheets receives UMMS Lifetime Achievement Award in Medical Education

2014	Dr. Skye is named director of Path of Excellence Program within new UMMS curriculum
2014	Appointment of Stephen M. Wampler, MD, as vice-chief of Medicine Service, Chelsea Community Hospital
2015	Dr. Skye is named one of four MHome learning community directors within new UMMS curriculum
2015	Caroline R. Richardson, MD, joins leadership team of Institute for Healthcare Policy and Innovation
2015	Dr. Ruffin is inducted into UMMS League of Research Excellence
2015	Ananda Sen, PhD, receives Collegiate Research Professorship Award
2015	Dr. Kiningham is awarded American Medical Society of Sports Medicine Founders' Award
2015	Dr. Zazove is featured on CNN's *The Human Factor*
2015	Initiation of Michael Papo, MD, Family Medicine Scholarship
July 2015	Initiation of Drs. Earl and Louise Zazove Lectureship in Family Medicine
2016	Initiation of Gazella-Brandle Memorial Family Medicine Scholarship
2016	Approval of Brighton Health Center
2016	Fourth associate chair for research programs: Dr. Richardson
2016	Second Dr. Max and Buena Lichter Research Professor of Family Medicine: Dr. Richardson
2016	Third associate chair of information management and quality (interim): Heather L. Holmstrom, MD
2016	Michael D. Fetters, MD, MPH, MA, serves as Fulbright Distinguished Chair of Social Sciences at Peking University Health Sciences Center
2016	Initiation of the Mixed Methods Research and Scholarship Program by Dr. Fetters and John W. Creswell, PhD
2017	Summer preceptorship formally is named the Kenneth and Judy Betz Summer Preceptorship
2017	First associate chair for population medicine (formerly Information Management and Quality): Kathryn M. Harmes, MD
2017	Approved expansion of residency class size to thirteen
2017	Announcement of move to 300 North Ingalls building
April 2018	Fortieth-year anniversary event

Appendices

Contents

Note: Data provided in appendices are through October 1, 2017.

Faculty List
1978 to Present

Name	Years
Terence C. Davies, MD	1978–90
R. Dale Lefever, PhD	1978–2006
Shirley A. McCormick, MD	1978–87
Harry E. Schneiter Jr., MD	1978–87
S. Margaret Davies, MD	1978–90
James F. Peggs, MD	1978–2014
Michael R. Liepman, MD	1979–82
Toni C. Antonucci, PhD	1979–97
Robert C. Weikart, DMin	1979–87
Suzanne C. Heller, ACSW	1979–83
Sarah A. Fox, EdD	1979–84
James F. McGloin Jr., PhD	1979–80
Jennifer E. Frank, MD	1980–83
Virginia L. Johnson, MD	1980–81
Charles B. Freer, MD	1980–83
Robert W. Reinhardt Jr., MD	1981–88
Leslie A. Shimp, PharmD	1982–2003
John M. O'Brien, MD	1982–
Kent J. Sheets, PhD	1982–
Warren R. Garr, MD	1982–88
Samuel E. Romano, PhD	1982–2017

Linda R. Cronenwett, PhD	1983–84
Jonathan G. A. Henry, MD	1983–84
Barbara S. Apgar, MD	1983–
Mindy A. Smith, MD	1983–96
Marian Cohen, ACSW	1983–2008
James C. Coyne, PhD	1984–2000
Chandice C. Harris, MSN	1984–88
Larry D. Roi, PhD	1984–86
Thomas L. Schwenk, MD	1984–2011
Ricardo G. Hahn, MD	1985–87
Caryl J. Heaton, DO	1985–89
Alan D. Weingrad, MD	1985–88
Lee A. Green, MD	1986–2012
Robert P. Vermaire, MD	1986–94
Lynn L. Swan, MD	1987–94
David R. Mehr, MD	1989–92
Mark M. Bajorek, MD	1989–91
Barbara D. Reed, MD	1989–2016
David J. Doukas, MD	1989–99
A. Evan Eyler, MD	1989–2002
Michael S. Klinkman, MD	1989–
Philip Zazove, MD	1989–
Mack T. Ruffin IV, MD	1990–2016
John D. Severin, MD	1990–99
Daniel W. Gorenflo, PhD	1990–2008
Martha O. Kershaw, MD	1991–2006
Ricardo R. Bartelme, MD	1991–2017
Raymond J. Rion, MD	1992–2002
Mark A. Zamorski, MD	1992–2001
Jennifer L. Hoock, MD	1992–98
Thomas R. Fahrbach, MD	1992–93
John T. Marquez, PhD	1993–97
Catherine A. Churgay, MD	1993–2002

Robert B. Kiningham, MD	1993–
Karen R. Fonde, MD	1993–2010
Michael D. Fetters, MD	1994–
Jean M. Malouin, MD	1994–
Pamela G. Rockwell, DO	1994–
Michael J. Worzniak, MD	1994–96
Jeffrey H. Sonis, MD	1994–2001
James R. Chenoweth, MD	1994–97
Adam C. Husney, MD	1994–95
Christine W. Krause, MD	1995–
Wayne A. Forde, MD	1995–97
Randall T. Forsch, MD	1995–
Steven G. Manikas, DO	1996–2000
Wendy S. Biggs, MD	1996–2002
Theresa R. Peters, MD	1996–
Michael L. Szymanski, MD	1996–2006
Elisa M. DeAngelis, MD	1996–97
Hector J. Llenderrozos, MD	1996–98
Patricia A. Marsh, MD	1996–2006
Randy K. Ward, MD	1996–2000
David J. Alvarez, DO	1996–
Toni M. Cutson, MD	1996–98
Jeffrey A. Housner, MD	1996–2001
Michelle L. Rabideau, MD	1996–
Stephen D. Elgert, MD	1996–99
William E. Chavey II, MD	1997–
John H. Affinito, MD	1997–2000
Kristina M. Gallagher, MD	1997–
Dawn E. Mooradian, MD	1997–2000
Eileen M. Reickert, MD	1997–2001
Deryth L. Stevens, MD	1997–2004
Mary P. Bassler, MD	1997–2003
Leon McDougle, MD	1997–2001

Matthew L. Denno, MD	1998–99
Kendalyn J. Murray, MD	1998–2002
Amy C. Miller, MD	1998–
Lourdes Velez, MD	1998–2016
Donald E. Nease Jr., MD	1998–2011
Phillip E. Rodgers, MD	1998–
Rita K. Benn, PhD	1998–2008
Suzanna M. Zick, ND	1998–
Kiyoshi Sano, MD	1999–2006
Joslyn M. Shehab, MD	1999–2006
Joyce E. Kaferle, MD	1999–2013
Eric P. Skye, MD	1999–
Geoffrey L. Jones, MD	1999–2001
Sara L. Warber, MD	1999–2016
Joel J. Heidelbaugh, MD	1999–
Mollie L. Kane, MD	1999–2002
Karen M. Kolias, MD	2000–2004
Karen L. Musolf, MD	2000–
James M. Cooke, MD	2000–
Linda K. Davenport, MD	2000–2001
Grant M. Greenberg, MD	2000–2016
Michele L. Pennington, MD	2000–2001
James E. Aikens, PhD	2000–
Caroline R. Richardson, MD	2001–
Tammara S. Stefanelli, MD	2001–2003
Elizabeth A. Dowell, MD	2001–2007
Amy B. Locke, MD	2002–2015
Uche D. George-Nwogu, MD	2002–
Tarannum A. Master-Hunter, MD	2002–
Seonae Yeo, PhD	2002–2007
Monica Myklebust, MD	2003–2007
Christine T. Cigolle, MD	2003–
David C. Serlin, MD	2003–

Stephen M. Wampler, MD	2003–
Ananda Sen, PhD	2003–
Jamie S. Weinstein, MD	2003–2007
Denise L. Campbell-Scherer, MD, PhD	2003–2008
Zora Djuric, PhD	2004–
Masahito Jimbo, MD, PhD	2004–
Janet L. Larsen, MD	2004–2007
Joy C. Williams, MD	2004–
Gary Yen, MD	2004–
Anne L. Kittendorf, MD	2004–
Catherine M. Bettcher, MD	2005–
Yosuke Fujioka, MD	2006–2009
Stefani A. Hudson, MD	2006–2015
Karl T. Rew, MD	2006–
Craig E. Ross, MD	2007–2009
Jill N. Fenske, MD	2007–
Elisa B. Picken, MD	2007–2017
Cheryl E. LaMore, MD	2007–
Kristy K. Brown, DO	2007–2011
Sahoko H. Little, MD, PhD	2008–
Scott A. Kelley, MD	2009–
Margaret A. Riley, MD	2009–
Heather L. Holmstrom, MD	2009–2017
Kathryn M. Harmes, MD	2009–
Katherine J. Gold, MD	2009–
Ebony C. Parker-Featherstone, MD	2010–
Keri L. Denay, MD	2011–
Margaret L. Dobson, MD	2011–
Jean H. Wong, MD	2011–
Abigail Lowther, MD	2011–2013
Alisa P. Young, MD	2011–
Laurie J. Legocki, PhD	2011–2013
Elizabeth K. Jones, MD	2012–

Thomas A. O'Neil, MD	2012–
Ghazwan Toma, MD	2012–
Mikel Llanes, MD	2012–
Elizabeth R. Shih, MD	2012–
Micheleen S. Hashikawa, MD	2012–
Nell B. Kirst, MD	2013–
Lorraine R. Buis, PhD	2013–
Tammy Chang, MD	2013–
Carissa A. Orizondo, MD	2013–
Christa B. Williams, MD	2013–
Michael M. McKee, MD	2013–
Weyinshet P. Gossa, MD	2014–2015
Amal Othman, MD	2014–
Ketti S. Petersen, MD	2014–
Jill R. Schneiderhan, MD	2014–
Christina A. Murphy, MD	2014–
Christina L. Chiang, MD	2015–
Allison N. Ursu, MD	2015–
Justine P. Wu, MD	2015–
Anita K. Hernandez, MD	2015–
Christine J. Medaugh, MD	2015–
Golfo K. Tzilos Wernette, PhD	2015–
Keturah P. Schacht, MD	2015–
Timothy C. Guetterman, PhD	2016–
Laura E. A. Heinrich, MD	2016–
Jenna B. Greenberg, MD	2016–
Anna K. Laurie, MD	2016–
Julie K. Prussack, MD	2016–
Angela L. Kuznia, MD	2016–
Ayano Kiyota, MD, PhD	2016–
Stephen J. Warnick, MD	2016–
Kevin M. Kuzia, MD	2017–
Elham Mahmoudi, PhD	2017–

Thomas W. Bishop, PsyD	2017–
Katherine E. Hughey, MD	2017–
Lydia U. Lee, MD	2017–
Lisa M. Meeks, PhD	2017–
Gregory D. Shumer, MD	2017–
Toshiaki Wakai, MD	2017–

Resident Graduates
1982 to 2017

1982
Scott Frank, MD
Patrick Kearney, MD
John O'Brien, MD
Fred Van Alstine, MD

1983
James Chenoweth, MD
Evelyn Eccles, MD
Thomas McRae, MD
James Meza, MD
Michael Sullivan, MD
Craig Weisse, MD

1984
Tama Abel, MD
Randy Baker, MD
James Dunlay, MD
Carole Tsou, MD
John Severin, MD
William Webb, MD
Susan Wentz, MD

1985
Thomas Hupy, MD
Michael Klinkman, MD
Robert McCurry, DO
Morris Moore, MD
Rosemary Pomponio,
    MD
Peter Zenti, MD

1986
Duff Bailey, MD
LuAnn Chen, MD
Lee Green, MD
Micki Kantrowitz, MD
Jeremiah Sable, MD
Robert Vermaire, MD

1987
Ann Eyler, MD
John Hallfrisch, MD
Christine Jerpbak, MD
Paul Lentz, MD
Dennis Lockrey, MD
Lynn Swan, MD

1988
Lawrence Frerker, MD
Susan Ivey, MD
Ellis Talbert, MD
Kevin Weber, MD
Elizabeth Wilson, DO

1989
Mark Bajorek, MD
Ruth Bosch, MD
Karl Edelmann, MD
Nadu Tuakli, MD
Paul Ward, MD

1990
Leslie Dale, MD
Mark Ebell, MD
Karen Eldevick, MD
Randall Forsch, MD
K. George Seifert, MD
Daniel Stulberg, MD

1991
Catherine Churgay, MD
Ronald Cotterel, MD
Thomas Fahrbach, MD
Lois Gregg, MD
Colleen Tallen, MD

1992
Susan Essman, MD
Anne Fitzpatrick, MD
Robert Kiningham, MD
Rose Ann Ng, MD

Lucy Runde, MD
Mark Zamorski, MD

1993
Paul Curtin, MD
Karen Fonde, MD
Joyce Koram, MD
Terri Maszatics, MD
Sami Rifat, MD

1994
Agatha Atko, DO
Lawrence Hall, MD
Adam Husney, MD
Joyce Kaferle, MD
Jean Skratek, MD
Jonathan Sorscher, MD

1995
David Alvarez, DO
William Chavey, MD
David Hirsh, MD
Christine Krause, MD
James Marsh, MD
Norine Tracy, MD
Richard Wynn, MD

1996
Mark Brumm, MD
Elisa DeAngelis, MD
Hector Llenderrozos, MD
Patricia Marsh, MD
Thomas Wang, MD

1997
John Affinito, MD
Chad Carlson, MD
Matthew Denno, MD
Kenneth Grimm, MD
Madhu Gupta, MD

Dawn Mooradian, MD
Dina Ozols, MD
Eileen Reickert, MD
Marian Ryan, MD
Sara Warber, MD

1998
William Borgos, MD
Nicole Cherbuliez, MD
Rebecca Moran, MD
Scott Paluska, MD
Phillip Rodgers, MD
Joslyn Shehab, MD
Melissa Sokol, MD
Jonna Whitman, MD

1999
Mona Ezzat, MD
Geoffrey Jones, MD
Mollie Kane, MD
Jon Lake, MD
Mona Merritt, MD
M. Sherwyn Mouw,
    MD
John Murry, MD
Marne Tower, MD
Amy Ullrich, MD

2000
Liberty Amador, MD
Kathleen Carr, MD
James Cooke, MD
Linda Davenport, MD
Grant Greenberg, MD
Vikrant Khanderia,
    MD
Brian Korte, MD
Tarannum Master, MD
Robert Nied, MD
Michael Schafer, MD

2001
Lorenzo Berlanga, MD
Roger Chen, MD
Chad Costley, MD
Karolyn Forbes, MD
Jun Ro, MD
Terry Samuels, MD
Shaunna Sears, MD
Tammara Stefanelli, MD
Dori Tamagne, MD
Adam Zolotor, MD

2002
Tanya Borisavljevic, MD
Jana Freed, MD
Jacqueline Friedman, MD
Amy Locke, MD
Tyra McKinney, MD
Esteban Miller, MD
Matthew Moore, MD
Jonathan Osburn, MD
Chadley Runyan, MD
Patricia Van Baren, MD

2003
Julia Bemer, MD
Jason Davenport, MD
Manjushree Deshpande, MD
Frederick Kron, MD
R. Karen Reiter, MD
Jennifer Schafer, MD
David Serlin, MD
Koryn Van Ittersum, MD
Stephen Wampler, MD
Jamie Weinstein, MD
Justine Wu, MD

2004
Darya Alexander, MD
Christopher Barnes, DO

Rajwinder Deu, MD
Kathryn Harmes, MD
Morteza Khodaee, MD
Anne Kittendorf, MD
David Lien, MD
Gary Yen, MD

2005
Catherine Bettcher, MD
Tamara Dennis, MD
Elise Georgi, MD
Katherine Gold, MD
Amanda Hallberg, MD
Harland Holman, MD
Curi Kim, MD
Mark Mirabelli, MD
Neilesh Shah, MD
Ramsey Shehab, MD

2006
Amy Blair, MD
Michael Bruderly, MD
David Feig, MD
Jill Fenske, MD
Stefani Hudson, MD
Erin Murfey, MD
Carrie Nicholson, MD
Naomi Pearsall, MD
Supak Sookkasikon, MD

2007
Andrea Breese, MD
Joseph Crow Jr., MD
Anne D'Alessandri, MD
Andrew Heyman, MD
Christine Kistler, MD
Michael McCartney, MD
Julie Phillips, MD
Elisa Picken, MD
Cheryl Strzoda, MD

Jean Wong, MD
David Yanga, MD

2008
Jamila Battle, MD
Susan Bettcher, MD
Andrew LaFleur, MD
James Lim, MD
Kassandra McGehee, MD
Tanika Pinn, MD
Margaret Riley, MD
John Stracks, MD
Carla Zahuranec, MD

2009
Jennifer Clem, MD
Laura Distel, MD
Miranda Huffman, MD
Scott Kelley, MD
Caroline King, MD
Hobart Lee, MD
Eric McLaughlin, MD
Ebony Parker-
    Featherstone, MD
Holly Ross, MD
Joshua Smith, MD

2010
Brian Bluhm, MD
Jillian Boroniec, MD
Tammy Chang, MD
Keri Denay, MD
Phuong Huynh, MD
Stephanie Kay, MD
Mikel Llanes, MD
Huong Tran, MD
Rachelle Wilcox, MD

2011
Marisyl de la Cruz, MD

Elizabeth Jones, MD
Jeffrey Kim, MD
Kei Miyazaki, MD
Thomas O'Neil, MD
Adaku Onyeji, MD
Suzanne Ross, MD
Jamie Szelagowski, MD
Alisa Young, MD

2012
Emily Brunner, MD
Jacob Bryan, MD
Michael Johansen, MD
Nell Kirst, MD
Michael Kopec, MD
Elizabeth Nguyen, MD
Jasmine Parvaz, MD, PhD
Puja Samudra, MD
Tyler Southwell, MD
Michelle Tortorello, MD
Kristi VanDerKolk, MD

2013
Ketti Augusztiny, MD
Heather Bidgoli, MD
Margaret Greenough, MD
Aaron Heindl, MD
Lindsey Kotagal, MD
Joanna Lee, DO
Christopher Love, MD
Christina Nisonger, MD
Keturah Schacht, MD
Audrey Van Weylan, MD

2014
Yasir Afzal, MD
John Breck, DO
Joanna Duquette, MD
Weyinshet Gossa, MD
Christina Li, MD

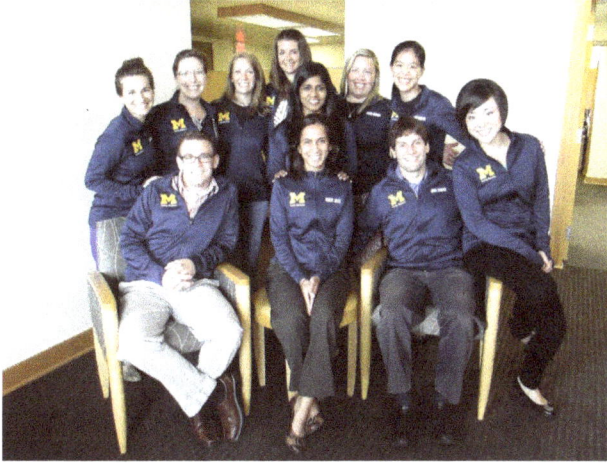

Figure B.1. Residency class of 2016 (July 2013)

Annelie Ott, MD
Ravishankar Rao, MD
Kathryn Shaffer, MD
Allison Ursu, MD

2015
Hetal Choxi, MD
Anthony Grech, MD
Jenna Greenberg, MD
Marisa Gross, MD
Amy Kreykes, MD
Anna Laurie, MD
Katherine Lemler, MD
Julie Prussack, MD

Belsam Saif, DO
Trevor Shull, MD
Kyle Smith, MD

2016
Kristine Cece, MD
Jane Chargot, MD
Andrew Cunningham, MD
Laura Heinrich, MD
Priyanka Kalapurayil, MD
Lydia Lee, MD
Heather McGovern, MD
Niyati Shah, MD
Gregory Shumer, MD

Katherine VanDrunen,
    MD
Angie Wang, MD

2017
Marian Deames, MD
Jacqueline Harrison, MD
Matthew Kittle, DO
Yuijing Lin, MD
Anna McEvoy, MD
Justin Oldfield, MD
Matthew Paletta, MD
Deborah Phipps, MD
Tyler Policht, MD

Appendix C

Recipients of Awards at Resident Graduation Ceremonies
1982 to 2017

Faculty Appreciation Senior Resident Award
Presented to the Faculty Member Who Best Typifies the Principles of Family Medicine in Character and Sensitivity to Resident Needs

1982	R. Dale Lefever, PhD	1997	James F. Peggs, MD
1983	Suzanne Heller, MSW	1998	Randall T. Forsch, MD
1984	John M. O'Brien, MD	1999	Randy K. Ward, MD
1985	Mindy A. Smith, MD	2000	John M. O'Brien, MD
1986	Robert W. Reinhardt, MD	2001	James F. Peggs, MD
1987	Barbara S. Apgar, MD	2002	Donald E. Nease Jr., MD
1988	Barbara S. Apgar, MD	2003	Mary P. Bassler, MD
1989	James F. Peggs, MD	2004	William E. Chavey II, MD
1990	Lynn L. Swan, MD	2005	Karen L. Musolf, MD
1991	James F. Peggs, MD	2006	Uche D. George-Nwogu, MD
	Robert P. Vermaire, MD	2007	Karen R. Fonde, MD
1992	Michael S. Klinkman, MD	2008	David C. Serlin, MD
1993	John D. Severin, MD	2009	Anne L. Kittendorf, MD
1994	Lee A. Green, MD	2010	Karen L. Musolf, MD
1995	Michael S. Klinkman, MD	2011	Kristy K. Brown, DO
1996	Catherine A. Churgay, MD	2012	Tarannum A. Master-Hunter, MD

2013	James M. Cooke, MD	2015	James E. Aikens, PhD
	Tarannum A. Master-Hunter, MD	2016	Karen L. Musolf, MD
2014	James M. Cooke, MD	2017	Elizabeth K. Jones, MD
	James F. Peggs, MD		

Resident Appreciation Award
For Encouragement and Assistance beyond the Call of Duty

1999	Wendy S. Biggs, MD	2010	Linda D. Lands
2000	Blythe A. Bieber		Deborah A. Wright
2001	William E. Chavey II, MD	2011	Mary E. Bieniasz, MS
2002	Barbara Gurd, RN	2012	Susan K. Guynn
2003	Blythe A. Bieber	2013	Susan E. Nehring, RN
2004	Eric P. Skye, MD	2014	Stacey S. Edman
2005	Jean E. Teifer		Suzanne B. McTaggert
2006	Samuel E. Romano, PhD	2015	Joel J. Heidelbaugh, MD
2007	Deborah A. Wright	2016	Katherine J. Gold, MD
2008	Linda D. Lands	2017	Margaret L. Dobson, MD
2009	Suresh Joshua, PA		

Award for Excellence in Teaching
In Recognition of Outstanding Contributions to Resident Education

1998	A. Evan Eyler, MD	2007	Barbara S. Apgar, MD
1999	Masahito Jimbo, MD	2008	Stephen M. Wampler, MD
2000	Phillip E. Rodgers, MD	2009	Masahito Jimbo, MD
	Eric P. Skye, MD	2010	Jeffrey A. Housner, MD
2001	Eric P. Skye, MD	2011	William E. Chavey II, MD
2002	John M. O'Brien, MD	2012	Uche D. George-Nwogu, MD
2003	James M. Cooke, MD	2013	Margaret L. Dobson, MD
2004	Grant M. Greenberg, MD	2014	Masahito Jimbo, MD, PhD
	Tarannum A. Master, MD	2015	Eric P. Skye, MD
2005	Pamela G. Rockwell, DO	2016	Ghazwan Toma, MD
2006	Joel J. Heidelbaugh, MD	2017	Karen L. Musolf, MD
	Janet L. Larsen, MD		

Thomas L. Schwenk, MD, Resident Teaching Award

**In Recognition of Demonstrated Interest, Ability, and
Commitment to Family Medicine Education**

1986	Lee A. Green, MD	2007	I. David Yanga, MD
1994	Adam C. Husney, MD	2008	Andrew M. LaFleur, MD
1998	Scott A. Paluska, MD	2009	Miranda McCann Huffman, MD, MEd
	Phillip E. Rodgers, MD		
1999	Geoffrey L. Jones, MD		Eric E. McLaughlin, MD
2000	Grant M. Greenberg, MD	2010	Jillian D. Boroniec, MD
2001	Not recorded	2011	Jeffrey L. Kim, MD
2002	Amy B. Locke, MD	2012	Elizabeth M. P. Nguyen, MD
2003	Manjushree Deshpande, MD	2013	Ketti S. Augusztiny, MD
2004	Not recorded	2014	Christina W. Li, MD
2005	Catherine M. Bettcher, MD	2015	Anthony S. Grech, MD
2006	Amy R. Blair, MD	2016	Gregory D. Shumer, MD
	Amanda J. Kaufman, MD	2017	Deborah A. Phipps, MD

Mack T. Ruffin IV, MD, MPH, Resident Original Project Award

**In Recognition of Demonstrated Interest, Ability, and
Commitment to Family Medicine Scholarship**

1992	Robert B. Kiningham, MD	2003	Jamie S. Weinstein, MD/Justine P. Wu, MD
1993	Not recorded		
1994	Jean M. Skratek, MD	2004	Christopher R. Barnes, DO/Rajwinder S. Deu, MD/Gary Yen, MD
1995	William E. Chavey II, MD		
1996	Not recorded		
1997	Not recorded	2005	Tamara S. Dennis, MD/Elise B. Georgi, MD/Curi Kim, MD
1998	Not recorded	2006	Amy R. Blair, MD/Stefani A. Hudson, MD
1999	Not recorded		
2000	Liberty B. Amador, MD/James M. Cooke, MD/Tarannum A. Master, MD/Michael W. Schafer, MD	2007	Julie P. Phillips, MD
		2008	Susan L. Bettcher, MD/Margaret A. Riley, MD
2001	Tammara S. Stefanelli, MD	2009	Caroline L. King, MD/Holly E. Ross, MD
2002	Tanya Borisavljevic, MD/Jana M. Freed, MD/Amy B. Locke, MD/Esteban E. Miller, MD	2010	Jillian D. Boroniec, MD/Phuong Nam-Thuy Huynh, MD/Rachelle Wilcox, MD

2011	Maria Syl D. de la Cruz, MD/Alisa P. Young, MD	2014	Alison N. Ursu, MD
		2015	Trevor W. Shull, MD
2012	Jacob J. Bryan, MD/Michelle L. Tortorello, MD	2016	Kristine L. Cece, MD/Jane E. Chargot, MD
	Nell Burger Kirst, MD/Elizabeth M. P. Nguyen, MD	2017	Deborah A. Phipps, MD
2013	Joanna T. Lee, DO		

Appendix D

Recipients of Awards and Scholarships at Award and Scholarship Ceremonies
1988 to 2017

Terence C. Davies, MD, Award

2017   Jennifer Jehnsen

Past recipients

2016	Julie A. Blaszczak	2006	Avani J. Sheth
2015	Grace P. Huang Amadi	2005	James F. Dolan
2014	Roshan F. Najafi	2004	Tracy K. Bozung
2013	Nathan D. Stern	2003	Michael I. Bruderly
2012	Justin Conway	2002	Te-Yu Ruth Chang
2011	Christina W. Li		Elise B. Georgi
2010	Ketti S. Augusztiny	2001	Anne L. Kittendorf
	Timothy A. Poulton	2000	Jameelah J. Gater
2009	Nell Burger Kirst	1999	Lisa M. Long
	David M. Lessens	1998	Stefani J. Day
2008	Matthew R. Meunier		Sonja N. Van Hala
	Suzanne V. Ross	1997	Grant M. Greenberg
2007	Tammy Chang	1996	Todd M. Shepard
	Stephen J. Warnick Jr.	1995	Scott A. Paluska

1995	Sharon K. Shepich	1991	David J. Gronski
1994	Mark J. Zawisa		Kim R. Kahler
1993	Diana R. Lewis	1990	Gerard A. Rudy
1992	Nicola J. Davies	1989	James Kerwin
	Thomas R. Graf	1988	Lisa J. Pierce

Department of Family Medicine Senior Scholarship

2017	Ross T. Avila

Past recipients

2016	Afrah Raza	2008	Elizabeth R. Meza
2015	Torrance C. Laury	2007	Crystal G. Kong
2014	David J. Gryniewicz	2006	Kevin M. Kuzia
2013	Julie K. Hubble	2005	Jennifer M. Dehlin
2012	Andrea Kussman	2004	Tracy T. Bozung
2011	Christina W. Li		Andrew H. Heyman
2010	Kimberly Vanderzee		

Harold Kessler, MD, Family Medicine Scholarship

2016–17	Nicole Castagno, Vikas K. Jayadeva, and Jennifer Jehnsen

Past recipients

2015–16	Kartik Sidhar,	2011–12	Hela Issaq
	Sarah A. Pettibone	2010–11	Jennifer J. Knoester
	Jonathan D. Waldmann	2009–10	Ketti S. Augusztiny
2014–15	Grace P. Huang Amadi	2008–9	David Lessens
	Harriet Huang	2007–8	Janani Krishnaswami
2013–14	Carson C. Phillips	2006–7	Tammy Chang
	Michael C. Vizachero	2005–6	Avani Sheth
2012–13	Nathan D. Stern	2004–5	Sarah Vanston

William Clippert Gorenflo Research Award in Family Medicine

2016–17	Julie A. Blaszczak, MD, and Jennifer N. Angell

Past award recipients

2015–16	Nicolas Johnson, MD	2010–11	Sara Bowling
	Kathryn Brown		Lindsay Davis
2014–15	Alissa D. Petrities	2009–10	Shawn Brown
2013–14	Hetal H. Choxi, MD	2008–9	Tammy Chang, MD
	Gregory D. Shumer, MD	2006–7	Julie P. Phillips, MD, MPH
2012–13	Weyinshet P. Gossa, MD	2005–6	Curi Kim, MD
2011–12	Joanna T. Lee, DO	2004–5	Katherine J. Gold, MD

Kenneth and Judy Betz Family Medicine Scholarship

2017   Jennifer Jehnsen

Past recipients

2016	Julie A. Blaszczak	2010	Ketti S. Augusztiny
2015	James Bailey	2009	Nell Burger Kirst
2014	Emily R. Torell	2008	Laura M. Breymann
2013	Nathan D. Stern	2007	Stephen J. Warnick Jr.
2012	Alexa R. Lindley	2006	Christine R. Westbrook
2011	Jennifer M. Brewer	2005	James F. Dolan

Dale L. Williams, MD, Family Medicine Scholarship

2017   Ellen B. Williams

Past recipients

2016	George R. Wasylyshyn	2012	Julie B. Kaplan
2015	David T. Schrock	2011	Allison Wessel
2014	Yujing Lin	2010	Audrey B. Richardson
2013	Andrew K. Cunningham	2009	Puja G. Samudra

Jill and Thomas R. Berglund, MD, Family Medicine Scholarship

2017   Rachel R. Bian

Past recipients

2016	Lindsey R. Kolar	2015	Shadia A. Yeihey

2014	Casey R. Graves	2011	Kristine E. Smith
2013	Yorgos E. Strangas	2010	Timothy A. Poulton
2012	Marisa E. Gross	2009	Tessa K. Dake

Chelsea Community Family Medicine Scholarship

2017   Ellen B. Williams

Past recipients

2016	Elizabeth M. Irish	2012	Anthony S. Grech
2015	David T. Schrock	2011	Annelie Ott
2014	Tyler L. Ladue	2010	Keturah P. Schacht
2013	Kristine R. Martel	2009	David M. Lessens

Vincent P. and Genevieve L. Burns Family Medicine Scholarship

2017   Miranda Velikoff

Past recipients

2016	Sarah A. Pettibone	2012	Sara A. Bowling
2015	Torrance C. Laury	2011	Katherine A. Christensen Belsky
2014	Susan F. Mead	2010	Caitlin E. Enright
2013	Nazneen F. Uddin	2009	David M. Lessens

AEI Sorority Family Medicine Scholarship

2017   Nicole Castagno

Past recipients

2016	Kartik Sidhar	2011	Allison Wessel
2015	Brittani M. Jackson	2010	Lindsey V. Kotagal
2014	Roshan F. Najafi		
2013	Kristine R. Martel		
2012	Jessica Guh		

Robert J. Fisher, MD, Family Medicine Scholarship

2017   Eric M. Spencer

Past recipients

2016	Dominic Kiley	2013	Andrew K. Cunningham
2015	Greg A. Jaffe	2012	Anthony S. Grech
2014	Tyler L. Ladue	2011	Matthew R. Schlough

Paddy and Donald N. Fitch, MD, Family Medicine Scholarship

2017   Vikas K. Jayadeva

Past recipients

2016	Jonathan D. Waldmann	2013	Angad P. Singh
2015	Marissa B. Lapedis	2012	Angeline Ti
2014	Michael C. Vizachero		

Michael Papo, MD, Family Medicine Scholarship

2017   Eric M. Spencer

Past recipients

| 2016 | Elizabeth M. Irish | 2014 | Camille M. Riddering |
| 2015 | Sofia Y. Ligard | 2013 | Yorgos E. Strangas |

Gazella-Brandle Memorial Family Medicine Scholarship

2017   Zeinab M. Rizk

Past recipient

2016   Jonathan D. Waldmann

Appendix E

Endowed Lectureships

Terence C. Davies, MD, Endowed Lectureship in Medical Education

The Terence C. Davies, MD, Endowed Lectureship in Medical Education supports an annual lectureship in family medicine, which will feature a prominent speaker and family medicine educator who embodies the same values and passion that Dr. Davies exemplified as Chair of the Department of Family Medicine (1978–86).

Presenter	Title	Date
Thomas L. Schwenk, MD *Dean, School of Medicine Vice President, Division of Health Sciences University of Nevada*	**Family Physicians as Leaders** (Inaugural Lecture)	October 8, 2014
Lee A. Green, MD, MPH *Professor and Chair Department of Family Medicine University of Alberta*	**Health Care in America: An Insider's Perspective From the Outside**	October 14, 2015
Daniel H. Pink *Author/Speaker*	**The Science of Motivation in Medicine, Education and Beyond**	November 9, 2016
Scott H. Frank, MD, MS *Director, Master of Public Health Program Case Western Reserve University School of Medicine*	**Principles for Authentic Population Health in Primary Care**	October 11, 2017

Drs. Earl and Louise Zazove Lectureship in Family Medicine

The Drs. Earl and Louise Zazove Lectureship in Family Medicine will support an annual lectureship in family medicine and an education program focused on aging that will feature a prominent speaker and family medicine educator.

Bernard Hammes, PhD
Director, Medical Humanities and Respecting Choices Gundersen Health System La Crosse, Wisconsin

How Advance Care Planning Can Improve Care (Inaugural Lecture)

July 22, 2015

Alon Y. Avidan, MD, MPH
Director, UCLA Sleep Disorders Center & UCLA Neurology Clinic University of California, Los Angeles, David Geffin School of Medicine Los Angeles, California

Sleep Disturbances in Older Age: What Lies Beneath?

July 13, 2016

Neelum T. Aggarwal, MD
Associate Professor, Department of Neurological Sciences and Alzheimer's Disease Center Rush University

Current Research Therapeutic Strategies for the Treatment and Prevention of Alzheimer's Disease

July 12, 2017

Appendix F

Department Leaders

Chairs

Terence C. Davies, MD, 1978–86

Thomas L. Schwenk, MD, 1986–2011

Philip Zazove, MD, 2011–Present

Chief Department Administrators

Francine M. Bomar, 1990–2005

Quinta Vreede, 2005–10

Matthew Bazzani, 2010–Present

Associate/Senior Associate Chair

James F. Peggs, MD, 1991–2014

Assistant Chair/Assistant Chair for Planning and Program Development

R. Dale Lefever, PhD, 1983–2006

Assistant/Associate Chair for Clinical Programs

Philip Zazove, MD, 1995–97

Raymond J. Rion, MD, 1997–2002

Jean M. Malouin, MD, MPH, 2002–13

David C. Serlin, MD, 2013–Present

Assistant/Associate Chair for Educational Programs

James F. Peggs, MD, 1995–2007

Eric P. Skye, MD, 2007–Present

Assistant/Associate Chair for Research Programs

Barbara D. Reed, MD, MPH, 1995–97

Lee A. Green, MD, MPH, 1997–2002

Mack T. Ruffin IV, MD, MPH, 2004–16

Caroline R. Richardson, MD, 2016–Present

Assistant/Associate Chair for Information Management and Quality

Lee A. Green, MD, MPH, 2006–12
Grant M. Greenberg, MD, 2012–16
Heather L. Holmstrom, MD, 2016–17
 (Interim)

Kathryn M. Harmes, MD, 2017–Present
 (Title Change to Associate Chair for
 Population Medicine)

Residency Directors

R. Dale Lefever, PhD, 1978–84
Thomas L. Schwenk, MD, 1984–86
John M. O'Brien, MD, 1986–2002

Eric P. Skye, MD, 2002–7
James M. Cooke, MD, 2007–13
Margaret L. Dobson, MD, 2013–Present

Service Chief

Terence C. Davies, MD, 1978–86
Thomas L. Schwenk, MD, 1986–2010

William E. Chavey II, MD,
 2010–Present

Medical Directors

Chelsea

Harry Schneiter, MD, 1978–80
James F. Peggs, MD, 1980–93
Lynn Swan, MD, 1993–95

Randall T. Forsch, MD, 1995–2005
Grant M. Greenberg, MD, 2005–13
Jill N. Fenske, MD, 2013–Present

Briarwood

Barbara S. Apgar, MD, 1986–90
A. Evan Eyler, MD, 1990–92
James R. Chenoweth, MD, 1992–93
Ricardo R. Bartelme, MD, 1993–96

Jean M. Malouin, MD, 1996–2008
David C. Serlin, MD, 2008–13
Ebony C. Parker-Featherstone, MD,
 2013–Present

Ypsilanti

Raymond J. Rion, MD, 1993–2000
Joel J. Heidelbaugh, MD, 2000–2007
Stefani A. Hudson, MD, 2007–14
Caroline R. Richardson, MD, 2014–16

Margaret A. Riley, MD, 2016–17
Stephen J. Warnick Jr., MD,
 2017–Present

Dexter

Michael L. Szymanski, MD, 1995–2002
Joyce E. Kaferle, MD, 2002–11

Kathryn M. Harmes, MD, 2011–Present

North East/East/Domino's Farms

Robert B. Kiningham, MD, 1995–98

Pamela G. Rockwell, DO, 1998–Present

Livonia

Elizabeth K. Jones, MD, 2014–Present

Closed Sites

Original Livonia (1997–2000)

Dawn E. Mooradian, MD

Stockbridge (1998–2000)

Deryth L. Stevens, MD

Appendix G

Fellowships

ACGME-Accredited Fellowships

Geriatric Medicine Fellowship (administered by Department of Internal Medicine), first family physician participated as a fellow in 1988

Sports Medicine Fellowship (administered by Department of Family Medicine), initiated in 1992, family physician participant in each year since initiation

Hospice and Palliative Care Medicine Fellowship (administered by Department of Internal Medicine), initiated in 2008, family physician participant in each year since initiation

Other Fellowships

Academic Fellowship (administered by Department of Family Medicine), initiated in 2006, family physician participant in each year since initiation

Integrative Medicine Fellowship (administered by Department of Family Medicine), initiated in 2007, family physician participant in each year since initiation

Women's Health Fellowship (administered by Department of Obstetrics and Gynecology), initiated in 2009, family physician participant in each year since initiation

2017 SODA Report Card
Department of Family Medicine, Thirty-Nine Years of Success

Department Characteristics			
Revenue	**2016 – 2017**	**99 Faculty/299 Staff** **33 Residents/12 Fellows**	**Total Revenue 1978 – 2017** **> $ 473.85 M**
Clinical	$ 15.6 M		
Grants/Contracts (Directs)	$ 3.3 M		
Institutional Support	$ 2.6 M	**Department Mission** *Increase the availability of quality primary health care to residents of the United States through the advancement and demonstration of the principles of family medicine as an academic discipline.*	
Philanthropy	$ .50 M		
Other	$ 1.9 M		
Total	**$ 24 M**		

Clinical Mission			
Outpatient Volume	**2016 – 2017**	**1978 – 2017**	**Total Outpatient Visits 1978 – 2017** **Approximately 3.2 M**
Briarwood (1986)	36,590	> 883,000	
Chelsea (1978)	30,565	> 1,066,000	
Dexter (1995)	20,796	> 299,000	**DFM Clinical Focus Measures** **(UMMG Performance/DFM Performance)**
Domino's (1993)	22,023	> 383,000	

			Clinical Focus Measures	Performance
Livonia (2014)	14,074	> 31,000	Adolescent Imms 2-Dose HPV by age 13 yrs – Males Females	47% / 43%
Ypsilanti (1993)	18,463	> 555,000	Advance Directive Documentation, >65 yrs – Adults	34% / 33% (75th %tile)
			Preventive Asthma - Adult Action Plan, Persistent Asthma	73% / 60% (75th %tile)
Total	**142,911**	**> 3,220,000**	Asthma – Adult Pneumococcal Vaccine, ALL Asthma	73% / 82% (75th %tile)
Inpatient Volume	**2016 – 2017**	**1978 – 2017**	Asthma – Pediatrics Action Plan, Persistent Asthma	90% / 84%
CFM	1,184	> 30,000	Depression Visit History – Use of PHQ-9, age > 12 yrs (visit encounter dx in past year)	49% / 55% (75th %tile)
UFM	1,384	> 20,000	Cervical Cancer Screening – Adults Preventive Care	
			Diabetes Adult – BP < 140/90	86% / 86% (75th %tile)
			Hypertension – BP Control (most recent BP)	76% / 78% (75th %tile)
				75% / 76% (75th %tile)
FMB	476	>10,900	**Total Inpatient Visits 1978 – 2017** **Approximately 73,600**	
FMN	514	> 11,000		
Total	**3,558**	**> 73,000**		

Educational Mission					
Predoctoral			**Residency**		
	2016 – 2017	**1978 – 2017**		**2016 – 2017**	**1978 – 2017**
Students Taught			Graduates		
M3	219	5,368	Residency	9	289
M4 (Elective/Sub I)	46		Academic	1	13
M3 Clerkship Ratings	1st for 18 out of 21 years!		Geriatric Medicine	1	30
Students Matching in FM	10.2% (17 out of 167)		Integrative Medicine	2	11
			Palliative Care	1	6
Continuing Medical Education			Sleep Medicine	1	4
			Sports Medicine	2	35
			Women's Health	2	12
			Individualized	1	2
	2016 – 2017	**1978 – 2017**	ABFM Board Examination Pass Rate		
Registrants	337	> 24,800	Our Residency (100%)		
Revenue	$ 140,817	> $ 23 M	National Pass Rate (95.9%)		
Average Rating	Exceeded/Met Expectations > 95%				
Total Educational RVUs for 2016 – 2017 17,192					

Research Mission		
	2016 – 2017	**1978 – 2017**
Research Grant Funding (Directs/Indirects)	$ 3,533,677	> $ 60 M
Grant Submissions	29	
% Capture of Family Medicine NIH Budget	4.61%	3.05%
Approximate NIH Ranking	6th	
Publications and Major Presentations	Hundreds!	Thousands!

Respect the elders	Play when you can	Share your affections
Teach the young	Hunt when you must	Voice your feelings
Cooperate with the pack	Rest in between	Leave your mark

Bequests Made to the University of Michigan Department of Family Medicine

Thank you to the following donors who have named the Department of Family Medicine in their estate plans. Total documented bequest giving is over seven million dollars.

- Elizabeth A. Burns, MD
- Joseph A. Caruso, MD
- Robert I. Cutcher, MD
- S. Margaret Davies, MD
- Terence C. Davies, MD
- Robert J. Fisher, MD
- J. William Fry, MD
- Daniel W. Gorenflo, PhD
- Bernard Kimmel, MD
- Leonora E. Nash-Morgan, MD, and John D. Morgan
- James F. Peggs, MD, and Margaret Talburtt, PhD
- Jane K. and Thomas L. Schwenk, MD
- Mary A. and William L. Smith, MD
- Sara L. Warber, MD
- Dale L. Williams, MD
- Earl Zazove, MD

Endowed Funds in the University of Michigan Department of Family Medicine

Professorships/Chairs

George A. Dean, MD, Chair of Family Medicine

Dr. Max and Buena Lichter Research Professorship

Endowed Lectureship

Terence C. Davies, MD, Lectureship in Medical Education

Drs. Earl and Louise Zazove Lectureship in Family Medicine

Endowed Scholarships

AEI Sorority Family Medicine Scholarship

Jill and Thomas R. Berglund, MD, Family Medicine Scholarship

Kenneth and Judy Betz Family Medicine Scholarship

Chelsea Community Family Medicine Scholarship

Department of Family Medicine Senior Scholarship

Robert J. Fisher, MD, Family Medicine Scholarship

Paddy and Donald N. Fitch Family Medicine Scholarship

Gazella-Brandle Memorial Family Medicine Scholarship

Harold Kessler, MD, Family Medicine Scholarship

Michael Papo, MD, Family Medicine Scholarship

Dale L. Williams, MD, Family Medicine Scholarship

Endowed Awards

Kenneth and Judy Betz M1/M2 Preceptorship Fund

Terence C. Davies, MD, Award

Karen R. Fonde, MD, Underserved Populations Fund

William C. Gorenflo Research Award

Mack T. Ruffin IV, MD, MPH, Resident Original Project Award

Thomas L. Schwenk, MD, Resident Teaching Award

Jane and Thomas L. Schwenk, MD, Faculty Award

Endowed Educational Funds

Alvin Johnson Stewart, MD, Fund

Spencer H. Wagar, MD, Fund

Sara L. Warber, MD, Health and Well-Being Education Endowment Fund

Other

Susan Guynn Residency Wellness Fund

Notes and Sources

Notes

Chapter 1

1 J. S. Millis et al., *The Graduate Education of the Physicians: The Report of the Citizens Commission on Graduate Medical Education* (Chicago: American Medical Association, 1966).

2 W. A. Willard et al., *Meeting the Challenge of Family Practice. Report of the Ad Hoc Committee on Education for Family Practice of the Council on Medical Education* (Chicago: American Medical Association, 1966).

3 Senate Concurrent Resolution No. 47, State of Michigan, Michigan Legislature. Adopted by the Senate, April 7, 1971, Adopted by the House of Representatives, May 14, 1971.

4 John A. Gronvall, MD, dean, University of Michigan Medical School, letter to Dr. J. Robert Willson, Dr. George Dean, Dr. Gary Gazella, Dr. Roland Hiss, Dr. Ramon Joseph, Dr. Charles Votaw, and Dr. Dale Williams, October 31, 1975.

5 University of Michigan Medical School (UMMS) Family Practice Residency Planning Committee Report, May 1976.

6 UMMS Family Practice Residency Planning Committee Report.

7 Daniel J. Ostergaard, MD, consultation report submitted to Charles L. Votaw, MD, PhD, January 21, 1977.

8 UMMS Family Practice Residency Planning Committee Report.

9 UMMS Family Practice Residency Planning Committee Report.

Chapter 2

1 Terence C. Davies, MD, University of Michigan Medical School Department of Family Practice Progress and Planning Overview, July 24, 1978.

2 University of Michigan Medical School Department of Family Practice Research Task Force Report, June 24, 1982.

3 Scott Frank, MD, Patrick J. Kearney, MD, John O'Brien, MD, and Fred Van Alstine, MD, open letter to the University of Michigan Department of Family Practice, June 23, 1982.

4 Terence C. Davies, MD, interview with the author, Virginia Beach, VA, August 7, 2015.

5 "Building on a Vision: Twenty Years of Family Medicine at the University of Michigan," brochure, University of Michigan, 1998.

6 "Building on a Vision."

7 "Building on a Vision."

8 "Department Enters New Era," *University of Michigan Department of Family Practice Alumni Society Newsletter* 2, no. 1 (Spring 1986).

9 Terence C. Davies, MD, "Reflections from the Chair," *University of Michigan Department of Family Practice Alumni Society Newsletter* 2, no. 1 (Spring 1986).

Chapter 3

1 Thomas L. Schwenk, MD, Department of Family Practice 1985–86 Annual Report.

2 John R. Wesley, MD, letter and report of the Family Practice Search Committee, submitted to Joseph E. Johnson III, MD, dean, University of Michigan Medical School, June 30, 1987.

3 Wesley, 1987.

4 Joseph V. Fisher, MD, "Remarks on the Occasion of the Tenth Anniversary of the Establishment of the Family Practice Department at the University of Michigan," speech, Decade of Caring Anniversary Event, Ann Arbor, MI, March 22, 1988.

5 "Julie A. Blaszczak Wins Top Department Award," *Family Medicine Newsletter*, Spring 2016.

6 Thomas L. Schwenk, MD, notes used in SODA presentation to the University of Michigan Department of Family Practice, December 4, 1991. The author has edited these remarks for length.

7 Thomas L. Schwenk, MD, email message to the author, January 27, 2016.

Chapter 4

1 A. Lorris Betz, MD, PhD, interim dean, University of Michigan Medical School, letter to Thomas L. Schwenk, MD, professor and chair, Department of Family Practice, September 16, 1996.

2 "Building on a Vision: Twenty Years of Family Medicine at the University of Michigan," brochure, University of Michigan, 1998.

3 "Building on a Vision."

4 Thomas L. Schwenk, MD, "Reflections from the Chair," *U-M Department of Family Medicine 1998 Fall/Winter Alumni Newsletter*.

5 "Building on a Vision."

Chapter 5

1 Dolores Goetz, The Wolf Credo, 1988.

2 Thomas L. Schwenk, MD, "The Department of Family Medicine: University of Michigan Medical School, 1978–2011," PowerPoint presentation to the Dean's Advisory Council of the University of Michigan Medical School, March 23, 2011.

Chapter 6

1 Philip Zazove, MD, written comments provided to the author to update information in the March 23, 2011, PowerPoint presentation to the Dean's Advisory Council of the University of Michigan Medical School, July 13, 2017.

2 R. Dale Lefever, PhD, email message to the author, October 4, 2017.

Chapter 7

1 Terence C. Davies, MD, University of Michigan Medical School Department of Family Practice Progress and Planning Overview, July 24, 1978.

2 Thomas L. Schwenk, MD, interview with the author, Reno, NV, January 14, 2016.

3 Philip Zazove, MD, interview with the author, Ann Arbor, MI, July 13, 2017.

4 "Building on a Vision: Twenty Years of Family Medicine at the University of Michigan," brochure, University of Michigan, 1998.

5 Letter from a patient to Elizabeth Jones, MD, September 8, 2017.

6 "2017 Student Scholarships & Awards," *Family Medicine Newsletter*, Summer 2017.

7 "The Future of Family Medicine: Student Scholarships & Awards Presented," *Family Medicine Newsletter*, Spring 2016.

8 "The Future of Family Medicine."

9 Thomas L. Schwenk, MD, "Reflections from the Chair," *Family Medicine Newsletter*, Spring 2011.

.

Sources

Given the nature of this book, most of the sources of information were not peer-reviewed publications or books. Most of the sources were letters, emails, and reports of various sorts. The most important sources were individuals who gave their time to be interviewed by the author or other colleagues. Not all these sources were cited in the notes, but the information gathered from each of these sources contributed to the overall content and context of the history of the University of Michigan Department of Family Medicine.

Interviews Conducted in Person by Kent J. Sheets, PhD

Terence C. Davies, MD, Virginia Beach, Virginia, August 7 and August 8, 2015
S. Margaret Davies, MD, Virginia Beach, Virginia, August 8, 2015
Patricia A. Warner, MPH, Ann Arbor, Michigan, September 29, 2015
Thomas L. Schwenk, MD, Ann Arbor, Michigan, October 13, 2015
Thomas L. Schwenk, MD, Reno, Nevada, January 14 and January 16, 2016
R. Dale Lefever, PhD, Ann Arbor, Michigan, March 17, 2016
Gary R. Gazella, MD, and Dale L. Williams, MD, Ypsilanti, Michigan, September 30, 2016
Daniel J. Ostergaard, MD, Leawood, Kansas, October 24, 2016
Peggy A. Campbell, Ann Arbor, Michigan, November 7, 2016
Philip Zazove, MD, Ann Arbor, Michigan, July 13, 2017

Interviews Conducted over the Telephone by Kent J. Sheets, PhD

C. Kent Smith, MD, November 2, 2016
Daniel J. Ostergaard, MD, January 18, 2017

Interviews Conducted in Person by Amy C. St. Amour

Marguerite R. Shearer, MD, Dexter, Michigan, June 28, 2017
Arlene B. Howe, Saline, Michigan, July 6 and July 13, 2017

Interview Conducted in Person by Rhian Davies-Hackenberg Using Questions Provided by Amy C. St. Amour and Kent J. Sheets, PhD

S. Margaret Davies, MD, Virginia Beach, Virginia, July 2017

Interview Conducted over the Telephone by

Amy C. St. Amour and R. Dale Lefever, PhD

George A. Dean, MD, January 2, 2017

Interview Conducted over the Telephone by Amy C. St. Amour

Nina I. McClelland, PhD, March 23, 2017

Personal Collections/Contributions

Terence C. Davies, MD

    A red three-ring binder labeled "Department of Family Practice. U of M. Ann Arbor. Papers
        Prior to March 1, 1978"

Thomas L. Schwenk, MD

    Box of reviews, annual reports, SODA notes, and other selected correspondence

Philip Zazove, MD

    Folder of printed email and other correspondence, SODA notes

Blythe A. Bieber

    Correspondence and other historical materials, hard copy and electronic

R. Dale Lefever, PhD

    Correspondence and other historical materials, hard copy and electronic

Kent J. Sheets, PhD

    Reports, training grants, correspondence, departmental newsletters, and brochures; artifacts
        bearing the department logo; and photographs

Miscellaneous Documents

Anniversary event brochures and programs

Internal and external review reports

Newsletters from 1985 to 2017

Residency brochures

Texts

Davenport, Horace W. *Not Just Any Medical School: The Science, Practice, and Teaching of Medicine at the University of Michigan, 1850–1941*. University of Michigan Press, 1999.

Frank, Scott. "Terry Davies: Permission to Become a Family Doctor." Unpublished essay.